Oncology at a Glance

This title is also available as an e-book.
For more details, please see
www.wiley.com/buy/9781118369692
or scan this QR code:

Oncology at a Glance

Graham G. Dark

MBBS, FRCP, FHEA
Senior Lecturer in Medical Oncology and Cancer Education
Department of Medical Oncology
Newcastle University
Freeman Hospital
Newcastle upon Tyne
UK

WILEY-BLACKWELL

A John Wiley & Sons, Ltd., Publication

This edition first published 2013 © 2013 by John Wiley & Sons, Ltd

Wiley-Blackwell is an imprint of John Wiley & Sons, formed by the merger of Wiley's global Scientific, Technical and Medical business with Blackwell Publishing.

Registered office: John Wiley & Sons, Ltd, The Atrium, Southern Gate, Chichester, West Sussex, PO19 8SQ, UK

Editorial offices: 9600 Garsington Road, Oxford, OX4 2DQ, UK
The Atrium, Southern Gate, Chichester, West Sussex, PO19 8SQ, UK
111 River Street, Hoboken, NJ 07030-5774, USA

For details of our global editorial offices, for customer services and for information about how to apply for permission to reuse the copyright material in this book please see our website at www.wiley.com/wiley-blackwell.

Library of Congress Cataloging-in-Publication Data

Dark, Graham
  Oncology at a glance / Graham G. Dark.
       p. ; cm. – (At a glance)
  Includes bibliographical references and index.
  ISBN 978-1-118-36969-2 (pbk. : alk. paper)
  I. Title. II. Series: At a glance series (Oxford, England)
  [DNLM: 1. Medical Oncology–methods.   2. Neoplasms–diagnosis.   3. Neoplasms–therapy. QZ 200]
  616.99'4–dc23

                                        2012044643

A catalogue record for this book is available from the British Library.

Wiley also publishes its books in a variety of electronic formats. Some content that appears in print may not be available in electronic books.

Cover image: Corbis
Cover design by Meaden Creative

Set in Times 9/11.5pt by Toppan Best-set Premedia Limited
Printed and bound in Malaysia by Vivar Printing Sdn Bhd

3   2016

Contents

Contributors

The following contributors were all medical students at Newcastle Medical School at the time of writing.

Attia Ahmed
Georgina Brehaut
Hayley Coleman
Joel Copperthwaite
Eleanor Earp
Katie Frampton
Rhiannon Hanson
Kamal Kaur
Kathryn Kelly
Elizabeth Kilcourse
Ashleigh Manning
Oliver Maunsell
Sarah Naisby
Osa Omosigho
Edward Rintoul
Amanda Rodrigues
Ross Sayers
Olivia Sharp
James Slack
Sam Small
Louise Thompson
George Walker

Preface

Oncology is a discipline that embraces a number of scientific fields. It is at the cutting edge of technology with regard to developments in therapeutic approaches. It is a stimulating and intellectual challenge to not only deliver the therapies of today but also to research and develop the treatments of tomorrow. Research is embedded within the specialties and reflects the origins within academic departments. The delivery of high-quality chemotherapy and radiotherapy services is an important political target and there has been considerable financial investment by the government in expanding cancer services in the UK.

For the undergraduate medical student oncology can be overwhelming, and often the exposure to patients with cancer can be quite fragmented in the undergraduate curriculum. Most student rotations will focus on the diagnostic processes as patients with cancer present to general medical and surgical firms, possibly as acute admissions or via outpatients with a variety of presenting symptoms. Other schools will provide specific rotations in the oncology department and this text is to provide the core knowledge to underpin such a learning experience.

The clinical practice of oncology is the application of a foundation of sciences, including: *anatomy*, to interpret radiological imaging; *physiology*, for the impact of a multisystem disease; *pharmacology*, to design, deliver and monitor systemic anticancer treatments; *molecular biology*, for the development of viable targets of therapy and to understand the mechanisms of carcinogenesis, genetic risk and resistance to therapy; *cell biology*, the process of metastasis, vascular invasion and microenvironment of the tumour and how this can affect outcome and approaches to therapy; *pathology*, to recognise the features of a disease that can affect all systems of the body.

Oncology is therefore the clinical application of the knowledge of science that underpins so much of clinical medicine and does so in an evidence-based manner. This requires clarity of understanding, a fastidious approach to investigation of the patient to obtain a diagnosis, and effective communication with the patient, their family and others within the multidisciplinary team. There are frequent challenges, as sometimes the investigations do not produce a definitive answer and yet a clear plan of management is required for the benefit of the patient.

For many, oncology seems like a depressing specialty and yet there is so much reward for those involved in the care of complex patients. The satisfaction of demonstrating clinical improvement after the intellectual challenge of getting the right diagnosis, planning the right treatment, given the context of the patient and their disease, having communicated understanding to the patient to explain what is likely to happen in the future and having had opportunity to address their concerns and fears, is a reward for many clinicians involved in the management of patients with complex problems, especially those with cancer.

The origins of **medical oncology** as a specialty lie in the management of haematological and paediatric malignancies. It began as a small research-oriented specialty and clinical research remains an important feature of the specialty. Over the past 20 years, enormous developments have taken place in the medical management of cancer, particularly in the development of therapies for the common solid tumours. Today, medical oncology is a broad-based clinical specialty. It ensures that for common cancers, state-of-the-art therapies of established efficacy are delivered on a national basis, within a framework of care, tailored for the patient as an individual. Medical oncologists increasingly see patients at the beginning of their cancer journey for consideration of adjuvant and neoadjuvant therapies. They work as part of a multidisciplinary team and are able to advise on all aspects of oncological treatment, including its integration with surgery and radiotherapy as well as having the skills to deliver specialist medical therapy.

Clinical oncology arose from the discovery of radiation and therapeutic irradiation, but most practitioners also deliver chemotherapy. In recent years there have been considerable technological advances in the delivery of radiation treatment with intensity modulation, photon therapy and stereotactic radiotherapy.

New anticancer treatments are constantly in development by clinicians who are working at the interface between the clinic and the scientific foundations of knowledge. There is therefore opportunity for individuals to develop an academic career as a clinician scientist with an interest in translational research that interfaces with the clinic.

This book is aimed at undergraduate students who will encounter patients with cancer throughout their clinical training and junior rotations. In some centres there may be minimal opportunity to study within the oncology departments because clinical experience may be gained with the teams that refer patients to a multidisciplinary team, rather than with the oncologists who deliver the subsequent treatment.

In some medical schools, students will have the opportunity to undertake a student-selected component (SSC). This is a period that allows personal learning outcomes to be defined and for individual students to explore either the depth or breadth of oncology practice. During one such period an informal discussion about learning resources resulted in the concept and idea of this book. A student focus group was used to identify the topics for inclusion and considerable attention was given to what is important for an undergraduate. Therefore some topics are left out by intention because they were not relevant to such an audience.

The SSC students were encouraged to research and write a chapter in an area of their own interest that reinforced their experience during the attachment. This project has allowed them to develop the skills of writing in a concise manner, while ensuring that the resulting text remained appropriate for the target audience. We are grateful to the student reviewers for their attention to detail and for providing constructive comments that have improved the content and allowed the project to remain focused.

This book is not a detailed reference text about cancer but instead has been written to provide a basic foundation of knowledge to underpin successful clinical training in cancer medicine for undergraduates of medicine and to provide an understanding of the principles of treatment approaches used for common cancers in oncology practice.

Graham G. Dark

Abbreviations

5-HIAA	5-hydroxyindoleacetic acid	**FNA**	fine-needle aspiration
5-HT	5-hydroxytryptamine (serotonin)	**G-CSF**	granulocyte-colony stimulating factor
5-HTP	5-hydroxytryptophan	**GCT**	germ cell tumour
ACTH	adrenocorticotrophic hormone	**GFR**	glomerular filtration rate
ADH	antidiuretic hormone or vasopressin	**GI**	gastrointestinal
AFP	alpha-fetoprotein	**GIST**	gastrointestinal stromal tumour
ALL	acute lymphoblastic leukaemia	**GU**	genitourinary
AML	acute myeloid leukaemia	**Gy**	Gray
ATP	adenosine triphosphate	**HAD**	hospital anxiety and depression scale
BCC	basal cell carcinoma	**HBV**	hepatitis B virus
BCG	Bacillus Calmette–Guérin	**HCC**	hepatocellular carcinoma
BMT	bone marrow transplant	**hCG**	human chorionic gonadotrophin
CACS	cancer anorexia and cachexia syndrome	**HCV**	hepatitis C virus
CD	cluster of differentiation	**HIV**	human immunodeficiency virus
CDK	cyclin-dependent kinase	**HNPCC**	hereditary non-polyposis colorectal cancer
CEA	carcinoembryonic antigen	**HOA**	hypertrophic osteoarthropathy
CHART	continuous hyperfractionated radiotherapy	**HPV**	human papilloma virus
CHRPE	congenital hypertrophy of the retinal pigment epithelium	**HRT**	hormone replacement therapy
CIN	cervical intraepithelial neoplasia	**HTLV-1**	human T-cell lymphotrophic virus-1
CINV	chemotherapy-induced nausea and vomiting	**ICP**	intracranial pressure
CIS	carcinoma in situ	**IDA**	iron-deficiency anaemia
CLL	chronic lymphocytic leukaemia	**IGF**	insulin-like growth factor
CML	chronic myeloid leukaemia	**IHC**	immunohistochemistry
CNS	central nervous system	**IL**	interleukin
COCP	combined oral contraceptive pill	**IMRT**	intensity-modulated radiotherapy
COX	cyclo-oxygenase	**IV**	intravenous
CR	complete response	**IVC**	inferior vena cava
CRP	C-reactive protein	**JVP**	jugular venous pressure
CSF	cerebrospinal fluid	**LCIS**	lobular carcinoma in situ
CT	computed tomography	**LCP**	Liverpool care pathway
CTC	common toxicity criteria	**LD**	longest diameter
CTZ	chemoreceptor trigger zone	**LDH**	lactate dehydrogenase
CUP	carcinoma of unknown primary	**LEMS**	Lambert–Eaton myasthenic syndrome
CVA	cerebrovascular accident	**LFT**	liver function tests
CXR	chest X-ray	**LHRH**	luteinising hormone-releasing hormone
DCIS	ductal carcinoma in situ	**MALT**	mucosa-associated lymphoid tissue
DLT	dose-limiting toxicity	**MDT**	multidisciplinary team
DNA	deoxyribonucleic acid	**MEN**	multiple endocrine neoplasia
DRR	digitally reconstructed radiograph	**mIBG**	meta-iodobenzylguanidine
DVT	deep vein thrombosis	**MR/MRI**	magnetic resonance imaging
EBV	Epstein–Barr virus	**MRCP**	magnetic resonance cholangiopancreatography
ECOG	Eastern Cooperative Oncology Group	**MSCC**	malignant spinal cord compression
EGFR	epidermal growth factor receptor	**MSU**	mid-stream urine
EM	electron microscopy	**MTD**	maximum tolerated dose
EMA	epithelial membrane antigen	**NER**	nucleotide excision repair
ENT	ear nose and throat	**NET**	neuroendocrine tumour
ER	oestrogen receptor/emergency room	**NHL**	non-Hodgkin's lymphoma
ERCP	endoscopic retrograde cholangiopancreatography	**NSAID**	non-steroidal anti-inflammatory drug
ESR	erythrocyte sedimentation rate	**NSCLC**	non-small cell lung cancer
eV	electron volt	**NSGCT**	non-seminomatous germ cell tumour
FAP	familial adenomatous polyposis	**OS**	overall survival
FBC	full blood count	**PCOS**	polycystic ovary syndrome
FDG	fluorodeoxyglucose	**PD**	progressive disease
FIGO	International Federation of Gynaecology and Obstetrics	**PDGF**	platelet-derived growth factor
FISH	fluorescent in-situ hybridisation	**PE**	pulmonary embolism

PEFR	peak expiratory flow rate
PEG	percutaneous endoscopic gastrostomy
PET	positron emission tomography
PFS	progression-free survival
PLAP	placental alkaline phosphatise
PMB	postmenopausal bleeding
PR	progesterone receptor/per rectum/partial response
PS	performance status
PSA	prostate-specific antigen
PT	prothrombin time
PTH	parathyroid hormone
PTHrP	parathyroid hormone-related polypeptide
PTT	partial thromboplastin time
PV	per vagina
RCC	renal cell carcinoma
RECIST	response evaluation criteria in solid tumours
RNA	ribonucleic acid
RR	relative risk
SCC	squamous cell carcinoma
SCF	supraclavicular fossa
SCLC	small cell lung cancer
SCT	stem cell transplant

SD	stable or static disease
SIAD	syndrome of inappropriate antidiuresis
SPECT	single photon emission computed tomography
SpR	specialist registrar
SVC	superior vena cava
TCC	transitional cell cancer
TENS	transcutaneous electrical nerve stimulation
TGF-α	transforming growth factor alpha
TGF-β	transforming growth factor beta
TLS	tumour lysis syndrome
TSH	thyroid-stimulating hormone
TURBT	transurethral resection of bladder tumour
TURP	transurethral resection of the prostate
TYA	teenager and young adult
U&E	urea and electrolytes
UMN	upper motor neurone
UTI	urinary tract infection
UV	ultraviolet
VAT	video-assisted thoracoscopy
VEGF	vascular endothelial growth factor
WHO	World Health Organization

1 The global burden of cancer

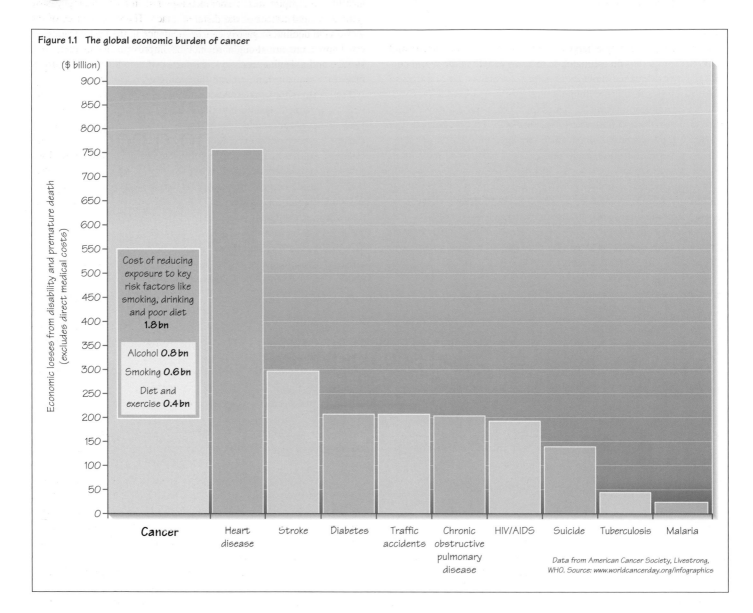

Figure 1.1 The global economic burden of cancer

Cost of reducing exposure to key risk factors like smoking, drinking and poor diet
1.8 bn

Alcohol **0.8 bn**

Smoking **0.6 bn**

Diet and exercise **0.4 bn**

y-axis: Economic losses from disability and premature death (excludes direct medical costs) — ($ billion)

x-axis categories: Cancer, Heart disease, Stroke, Diabetes, Traffic accidents, Chronic obstructive pulmonary disease, HIV/AIDS, Suicide, Tuberculosis, Malaria

Data from American Cancer Society, Livestrong, WHO. Source: www.worldcancerday.org/infographics

The global burden of cancer

Cancer represents a significant economic burden for the global economy and is now the third leading cause of death worldwide. By 2030, it is projected that there will be 26 million new cancer cases and 17 million cancer deaths per year.

The developing world is disproportionately affected by cancer, and in 2008, developing nations accounted for 56% of new cancer cases and 75% of cancer deaths. These deaths happen in countries with limited or no access to treatment and with low per capita expenditure on healthcare. In recognition of this, the Union for International Cancer Control conceived the World Cancer Declaration in 2009 to achieve 11 targets by 2020.

World Cancer Declaration

1. Sustainable cancer care delivery in all countries
2. Measurement and monitoring of the global cancer burden
3. Reduce global tobacco and alcohol use, and obesity
4. Universal hepatitis B and HPV vaccination
5. Improve the public's understanding of and attitude towards cancer
6. Screening and early detection programmes
7. Access to cancer services, including diagnosis, rehabilitation and palliation
8. Universal pain control
9. Increased training opportunities for healthcare workers
10. Reduce emigration of specialist cancer healthcare workers
11. Improvements in cancer survival

Developed and developing countries

Developing nations do not have the funding, expertise or infrastructure to deliver effective cancer services. They have limited or no cancer screening, few facilities and patients have limited access to treatments and analgesia. The lowest-income countries have a survival rate of

25%, compared with 56% in the wealthiest. Prevention is therefore a key strategy to reduce cancer deaths as it has the largest potential impact at the least expense.

Tobacco

Tobacco use is the single largest preventable cause of cancer and premature death, and an estimated 1.3 billion people in the world currently smoke tobacco. Smoking prevalence is highest among men in Eastern Europe, the former Soviet Union, China and Indonesia. Cigarette smoking among women has been decreasing in most high-resource countries but is stable or increasing in several countries in Southern, Central and Eastern Europe. With declining tobacco usage in many industrialised countries, the popularity of smoking has shifted to the developing world, especially for men.

Tobacco contributes to the development of 3 million cancers (lung, oropharynx, larynx, bladder and kidney), which could be prevented by smoking cessation. Lung cancer has been the most common cancer in the world since 1985 and cigarette smoking accounts for more then 20% of all global cancer deaths, 80% of lung cancer cases in men and 50% of lung cancer cases in women worldwide.

Lifestyle

Like tobacco, obesity, physical inactivity and poor nutrition are established causes of several types of cancer. Diet contributes to 3 million cancer deaths per year (gastric, colon, oesophagus, breast, liver, oropharynx and prostate); diet modification – avoiding animal fat and red meat, increasing fibre, fresh fruit and vegetable intake, as well as avoiding obesity – could reduce these.

A significant increase in the incidence of obesity (body mass index greater than 30 in adults) has occurred globally since the 1980s. The trend towards overweight and obesity is even greater in children than in adults and has occurred not only in high-resource countries but also in urban and even rural areas of many low- and middle-income countries. This is attributed to increased availability of calorie-dense foods and reduced physical activity.

Infections

Chronic infection accounts for 18% of cancers worldwide, the most common including cancers of the cervix, stomach and liver, in turn caused by HPV, *Helicobacter pylori* and hepatitis B and C virus. These pathogens are more prevalent in developing nations, where the resulting cancers are threefold more prevalent (26% compared with 8% in developed nations).

Cervical cancer is the fourth leading cause of cancer mortality in women worldwide, with 80% of cases in developing nations. HPV infection rates can be reduced by the use of condoms, and in more recent years a vaccination against HPV has become available. Rwanda became the first country in Africa to introduce HPV vaccination and screening for cervical cancer following donations by pharmaceutical and diagnostic companies.

The incidence and death rates from gastric cancer have steadily declined over the past 50 years, even though it remains the second leading cause of cancer mortality (65% in developing nations). Chronic or recurrent infection with *H. pylori* is the main cause of chronic gastritis and peptic ulcers and increases risk for developing gastric lymphoma and cancer of the distal stomach. The exact causes of the worldwide decline in gastric cancer incidence in the past decades are not known but are thought to include improvements in diet, food storage and a decline in *H. pylori* infection due to a general improvement in sanitary conditions and increasing use of antibiotics.

More than 80% of liver cancer cases occur in developing nations, with more than 55% occurring in China alone. Globally, 75% of all liver cancer cases and 50% of all deaths are caused by chronic infection with either HBV or HCV. A safe and effective vaccine against HBV is available and is the most cost-effective strategy to reduce liver cancer. More than three-quarters of WHO member states have introduced hepatitis B vaccine into routine infant immunisation schedules, although vaccine delivery is particularly challenging in high-risk, low-resource areas of Africa.

Challenges

Prevention with vaccination against certain cancers could reduce the cancer burden, with protection against HBV and HPV.

Education is important as low rates of literacy are associated with regions of poverty. Education about cancer could result in earlier diagnosis, better engagement with screening, and acceptance of diagnostic and treatment services. Such approaches need to reflect the local cultural requirements.

Access to treatment is resource limited as treatment for cancer relies on surgery, radiotherapy and chemotherapy, all of which remain expensive and often unavailable in developing nations. New targeted therapies will be too expensive and therefore the newest developments in therapy will be unavailable without successful engagement of the pharmaceutical industry to negotiate reimbursement schemes that might make new drugs more affordable and accessible.

Cure the curable: with a greater understanding of the hallmarks of cancer, specific features of cancers can be used as targets for treatment and could be used to reclassify the cancers. Understanding the microenvironment of the cancer cell is vital to delivering successful future therapies, but open access to research findings for all nations should be a key principle for funding research.

Provide palliation whenever it is required as the majority of cancer treatment is not aimed at cure, but more to control the patient's symptoms. Access to analgesia is often poor, with only 9% of the world's morphine used in developing nations, which have 83% of the world's population. In some regions of Africa, patients have to walk for more than a day in each direction to and from a pharmacy to receive only 5 days' supply of medication. There are persisting misconceptions about the problems of strong opioid analgesia that have yet to be overcome.

End of life care is not expensive but requires involvement of the family and other care givers. It can be improved by access to better training and education and provision of community-based services that understand the diversity and requirements of the local population.

2 The nomenclature of oncology

Table 2.1 Nomenclature of tumours

Originating tissue	Benign tumour	Malignant tumour
Blood vessel	Angioma	Angiosarcoma
Bone	Osteoma	Osteosarcoma
Cartilage	Chondroma	Chondrosarcoma
Fat	Lipoma	Liposarcoma
Fibrous tissue	Fibroma	Fibrosarcoma
Germ cell	Mature teratoma/dermoid cyst	Immature teratoma Seminoma/dysgerminoma
Glandular epithelium	Adenoma	Adenocarcinoma
Granulocyte		Myeloid leukaemia
Liver	Hepatic adenoma	Hepatocellular carcinoma
Marrow lymphocyte		Lymphocytic leukaemia
Node lymphocyte		Lymphoma
Plasma cell		Malignant myeloma
Skin	Papilloma	Squamous cell carcinoma Basal cell carcinoma
Skin melanocyte	Naevus	Malignant melanoma
Smooth muscle	Leiomyoma	Leiomyosarcoma
Squamous epithelium	Squamous papilloma	Squamous cell carcinoma
Striated muscle	Rhabdomyoma	Rhabdomyosarcoma
Transitional epithelium	Transitional papilloma	Transitional cell carcinoma

Table 2.2 Eastern Cooperative Oncology Group (ECOG) performance status scale

Score	Description
0	Fully active, able to carry out normal activities without restriction and without the need for analgesics
1	Restricted in strenuous activity, but ambulatory and able to carry out light work or pursue a sedentary occupation. This group also includes patients who are fully active but only with the aid of analgesics
2	Ambulatory and capable of self-care but unable to work Up and about for more than 50% of waking hours
3	Capable only of limited self-care Confined to a bed or chair for more than 50% of waking hours
4	Completely disabled Unable to carry out any self-care and permanently confined to a bed or chair

Table 2.3 Karnofsky performance status scale

Score (%)	Description
100	Normal, no complaints, no evidence of disease
90	Able to carry on normal activity, minor signs or symptoms
80	Normal activity with effort, some signs or symptoms
70	Cares for self, unable to carry on normal activity or do active work
60	Requires occasional assistance, but able to care for most of needs
50	Requires considerable assistance and frequent medical care
40	Disabled, requires special care and assistance
30	Severely disabled, hospitalisation indicated but death not imminent
20	Very sick, hospitalisation required, active supportive treatment required
10	Moribund, fatal processes progressing rapidly

The diagnosis of cancer is usually made following a histological assessment of a biopsy or resected specimen. The results should be interpreted within the context of the clinical case and discussed at a multidisciplinary meeting involving oncologists and the pathologist. The histopathological features of cancer include: abnormal cellular morphology, increased rate of mitosis, multinucleated cells, increased nuclear DNA and nuclear to cytoplasmic ratio, and tissue architecture that is less organised than that of the originating tissue. A histopathology report will outline the gross features (tumour size, lymph node size and number) and microscopic findings (tumour grade, margins, lymphovascular invasion, mitotic rate, immunohistochemistry staining).

Tumours typically invade the basement membrane, but those that have not yet done so are termed *in situ* tumours. These are non-invasive but demonstrate all the other features of cancer. They represent a stage in the progression from dysplasia to cancer.

Tumour nomenclature

The suffix *-oma* (Greek, 'swelling') is used to denote a benign tumour, although some are not tumours (e.g. granuloma). If the tumour is malignant the suffix *-carcinoma* (Greek, 'crab') is used for epithelial tumours and *-sarcoma* (Greek, 'flesh') is used for tumours derived from connective tissue. Table 2.1 outlines the common terms used for benign and malignant tumours arranged by originating tissue.

Prefixes are used to denote the originating tissue of the tumour, e.g. *adeno-* for glandular epithelium, *osteo-* for bone, *lipo-* for fat, *angio-* for vasculature, etc. The four main originating tissues are: epithelial tissue; connective tissue; lymphoid and haemopoietic tissue; and germ cells. Germ cell derivatives use the term *terato-* (Greek, 'monster'). Other tumours, because of prolonged usage, continue to bear eponyms (e.g. Hodgkin's disease, Kaposi sarcoma).

Sometimes there is more than one type of cancer tissue present within a single organ (e.g. carcinosarcoma) or within a single type of epithelium (e.g. adenosquamous carcinoma), each with its own special characteristics, prognosis and response to therapy. In some epithelial cancers the cancer tissue may not fit within a known classification and is often termed carcinoma NOS ('not otherwise specified').

Tumour grade

Tumours are graded by the degree of differentiation and growth rate, often on a scale of 1 to 3, where 3 represents the least differentiated, fastest-dividing tumours. Tumours that more closely resemble the tissue of origin are graded as well-differentiated (grade 1), while tumours with a more aggressive growth and high mitotic rates are graded as poorly differentiated (grade 3) cancers. The term anaplastic (Greek, 'to form backwards') is used to describe tumours that are so poorly differentiated that they have very few tissue-specific features and often do not stain well to surface markers.

The grade has prognostic significance, with grade 1 tending to have a more favourable prognosis and grade 3 the worst. Formal grading systems exist for a range of cancers but it does remain a subjective assessment, and typically a single cancer can be heterogeneous such that areas differing significantly in differentiation and mitotic activity exist side by side, with a risk of sampling error. Therefore for accurate diagnosis and grading, sufficient tissue and microscopic sections must be sampled so that the most malignant areas are found.

Some cancers are so well differentiated that their malignant cells cannot be distinguished from those of benign tumours or even from normal cells. In such instances, the recognition of abnormal cellular relationships becomes especially important for correct diagnosis.

Cytology

The examination of cells can be useful for a diagnosis in patients who have had a fine-needle aspiration (FNA) of a palpable mass. Fluid cytology can be performed on ascites, pleural fluid or CSF and can be diagnostic in some cases. However, sampling errors can lead to false-negative results whereas active infection or abscess formation may produce false-positive results. Cytology can examine cells from sputum, urine, the cervix, pleural effusions and ascites.

Abnormalities of individual cancer cells may be helpful in diagnosis, particularly increased numbers of mitoses and cytological features relating to the state of tumour cell differentiation. Cytological features of malignancy include altered polarity, tumour cell enlargement, increased nuclear to cytoplasmic ratio, pleomorphism (variation in size and shape) of tumour cells and their nuclei, clumping of nuclear chromatin and distribution of chromatin along the nuclear membrane, enlarged nucleoli, atypical or bizarre mitoses (e.g. tripolar) and tumour giant cells with one or more nuclei.

Cytogenetic analysis

Some tumours have typical chromosomal changes that can aid diagnosis and these specific abnormalities are usually demonstrated using a karyotype. In karyotype nomenclature, 9q31 designates the chromosome (9), the long arm (q) (rather than the short arm [p]), the region distal to the centromere (3) and the band within that region (1). The utilisation of fluorescent in-situ hybridisation (FISH) techniques can be useful in specific cancers, such as Ewing's sarcoma, and peripheral neuroectodermal tumours where there is a translocation between chromosome 11 and 22 – t(11; 22)(q24; q12).

Tumour stage

The stage of a cancer is a geographical term that denotes the extent of tumour spread, and a uniform classification system is used based on the size of the primary tumour (T), the presence of involved lymph nodes (N) and distant metastases (M). The TNM classification varies between different tumour sites and some cancers have different approaches (e.g. FIGO in ovarian cancer; Ann Arbor in lymphoma).

Performance status

One of the most important factors that impacts on the planning of treatment and prognosis is the performance status of the patient. This requires an assessment of their functional capacity, ability to self-care and mobility. The performance status correlates with prognosis and tolerance of treatment and a number of different scales are used, the more common being the ECOG (Table 2.2) and Karnofsky scales (Table 2.3).

Patients with performance status 3 or 4 do not tolerate treatment as well as those with performance status 0, 1 or 2, and indeed some systemic chemotherapy may shorten their life.

3 Environmental determinants of cancer

Table 3.1 Environmental influence on carcinogenesis

Factor	Processes	Cancers associated
Occupational exposure (see also Ultraviolet and Radiation)	Dye and rubber manufacturing (aromatic amines)	Bladder cancer
	Asbestos mining, construction work, shipbuilding (asbestos)	Lung cancer, mesothelioma
	Hardwood furniture making (hardwood dust)	Nasal cavity adenocarcinoma
	Vinyl chloride manufacturing (PVC)	Liver angiosarcoma
	Petrochemical industry (benzene)	Acute leukaemia
Chemicals	Chemotherapy (e.g. melphalan, cyclophosphamide)	Acute myeloid leukaemia
	Pesticide manufacture and copper refining (arsenic)	Lung cancer, squamous cell skin cancer
Cigarette smoking	Exposure to carcinogens from inhaled smoke	Lung cancer, bladder cancer
Viral infection	Herpes viruses (EBV, HHV-8)	Burkitt's lymphoma, nasopharyngeal cancer, Kaposi's sarcoma
	Hepatitis viruses (HBV, HVC)	Hepatocellular carcinoma
	Retroviruses (HTLV-1)	Adult T-cell leukaemia
	Papilloma viruses (HPV)	Cervical cancer, anal cancer
Bacterial infection	Helicobacter pylori	Gastric cancer, gastric mucosa-associated lymphoid tissue (MALT) lymphomas
Parasitic infection	Liver fluke (Opisthorchis sinensis)	Cholangiocarcinoma
	Schistosoma haematobium	Squamous cell bladder cancer
Dietary factors	Low roughage/high fat content diet	Colorectal cancer
	High nitrosamine intake	Gastric cancer
	Aflatoxin from contamination of Aspergillus flavus	Hepatocellular cancer
Radiation	Ultraviolet (UV) exposure	Basal cell carcinoma, melanoma, non-melanocytic skin cancer
	Nuclear fallout following explosion (e.g. Hiroshima)	Leukaemia, solid tumours
	Diagnostic exposure (e.g. CT imaging)	Cholangiocarcinoma (following thorotrast usage)
	Occupational exposure (e.g. Beryllium and strontium mining)	Lung cancer
	Therapeutic radiotherapy	Medullary thyroid cancer, sarcoma
Inflammatory diseases	Ulcerative colitis	Colon cancer
Hormonal	Androgenic anabolic steroids	Hepatocellular carcinoma
	Oestrogens	Endometrial cancer, breast cancer

Table 3.2 Effects of hormone manipulation on cancer risk

	Combined oral contraceptive	Hormone replacement therapy	Nulliparity and low parity
Ovarian cancer	Reduced risk	Increased risk (small)	Increased risk
Breast cancer	No effect	Increased risk	Increased risk
Endometrial cancer	Reduced risk	Increased risk if oestrogen only	Increased risk

Environmental factors

The majority of cancers result from a complex interaction between genetic factors and exposure to environmental carcinogens. Most of these environmental triggers have been identified using epidemiological studies which examine patterns of cancer distribution in patients of different age, sex, social class, geography, with different concomitant illnesses (Table 3.1). Sometimes these give strong pointers to the molecular or cellular causes of the disease, but for many solid cancers there is evidence of a multifactorial pathogenesis even when there is a known principal cause.

Radiation

The major physical carcinogen is radiation, which is ubiquitous in the environment and may be ionising or non-ionising. Ionising radiation is very high-energy radiation and includes gamma rays from cosmic radiation, isotope decay such as alpha particles from radon gas, and X-rays from medical imaging. Non-ionising radiation has less energy and includes ultraviolet radiation from the sun and radiofrequency radiation from electronic devices.

High-frequency, high-energy ionising radiation damages cellular structures and DNA by displacing electrons from atoms, resulting in an ion pair. Some tissues, such as bone marrow, thyroid and breast tissue, are particularly susceptible to the effects of ionising radiation.

Non-ionising radiation does not yield an ion pair but can still excite electrons, resulting in a chemical change to the target tissue. It is UVB that is the most significant in this category. However, UVC has the most potent effect on DNA, but it is quickly absorbed in air, making its effects negligible. Distortion of the DNA double helix results from a thymidine dimer that produces covalent bonding of adjacent thymidine residues on the same DNA strand. This distortion is normally repaired by the nucleotide excision repair (NER) pathway. Patients with xeroderma pigmentosum have defects in this mechanism, resulting in UV-induced skin malignancies. The incidence of cancers is greater in less pigmented populations because melanin absorbs UV radiation and acts to shield the dividing cells in the skin. Severe sunburn in youth is a significant risk factor for the subsequent development of malignant melanoma.

Chemicals

Many chemicals can induce cancer and are referred to as carcinogens, which can act on three distinct steps of initiation, promotion and progression. Initiation requires replication of cells where repair of the chemically induced DNA damage has failed, and a single exposure to a carcinogen may be sufficient. Promotion is a reversible process requiring multiple exposures, often with a dose-response threshold, which produces a selective growth advantage, usually without DNA mutation. Progression is irreversible and involves multiple complex DNA changes, such as chromosomal alterations and morphological cellular changes, which are detectable with microscopy.

Many potent carcinogens are strong electrophiles that can accept electrons, such as vinyl chloride, aflatoxin, N-hydroxylated metabolites of azo dyes and alkyldiazonium ions from nitrosamines.

Smoking

The chemical constituents of tobacco smoke are carcinogens and particularly increase the risk of lung, oropharyngeal, oesophageal and bladder cancers. However, associations exist with all cancers, with the exception of endometrial cancer for which smoking appears to be protective. Ninety per cent of lung cancers are directly attributable to smoking, and mortality from lung cancer is 30-fold higher in smokers than in non-smokers. Inhalation of mainstream smoke is most associated with cancer, but passive smoking will increase risk significantly.

Infections

Infection makes the most significant contribution to the global burden of cancer, with approximately 1.5 million cases of cancer (15%) per year (cervical, stomach, liver, bladder and lymphoma) due to infection. The association between virus infection and cancer was first demonstrated in 1911 by Peyton Rous, studying the development of sarcoma in chickens. Following HIV infection, the weakened immune system cannot respond to other viral carcinogens. In the presence of HIV, those infected with human herpes virus (HHV) 8 will develop Kaposi's sarcoma and Castleman's syndrome. The majority of other herpes viruses have been implicated in cancers, most notably Epstein–Barr virus (EBV) in causing Hodgkin's lymphoma or Burkitt's lymphoma.

The papilloma viruses HPV 16, 18, 31 and 45 are major aetiological factors for the development of cervical cancer, and the hepatitis B and C viruses are known causes of hepatocellular carcinoma. The main parasitic infections linked to cancer are malaria associated with Burkitt's lymphoma and schistosoma associated with various other cancers. Schistosoma japonicum has been linked to colorectal, hepatocellular and lymphoreticular cancers, and schistosoma haematobium to bladder cancer. Chronic inflammation is thought to play a central role in both cases. Chronic bacterial infections such as tuberculosis have been linked to an increased risk of developing cancer.

Hormones

Cancer can be induced by overproduction of endogenous hormones as well as exogenous substances as contained within the combined oral contraceptive pill (COCP) and hormone replacement therapy (HRT) (Table 3.2). Risk of breast cancer is related to the duration of exposure to oestrogens, with risk increased by low parity, early menarche, late menopause and prolonged exposure to oestrogens by the use of HRT. The COCP does not increase risk as it is used at a time in the life cycle when oestrogen is naturally present. Ovarian cancer is related to the number of ovulations, therefore the risk is increased by nulliparity but reduced by the COCP, reducing by 50% in those taking the COCP for 10 or more years. The risk of endometrial cancer in postmenopausal women is increased by using oestrogen-only HRT or tamoxifen.

Nutrition and lifestyle

Around 30% of all cancers and up to 70% of gastrointestinal (GI) malignancies are thought to be associated with poor nutrition, and obesity increases the risk of cancer, independent of quality of diet. Alcohol is associated with cancers of the GI tract, liver, breast and ovary, possibly by causing oxidative stress and prolonged exposure to acetaldehyde, the main metabolite of alcohol. Patients with alcohol-induced liver cirrhosis are at increased risk of hepatocellular carcinoma. Lifestyle changes can impact on risk; for example, the risk of breast cancer in women of Far Eastern origin remains relatively low when they first migrate to a country with a Western lifestyle, but rises in subsequent generations to approach that of the resident population of the host country.

4 The hallmarks of cancer I

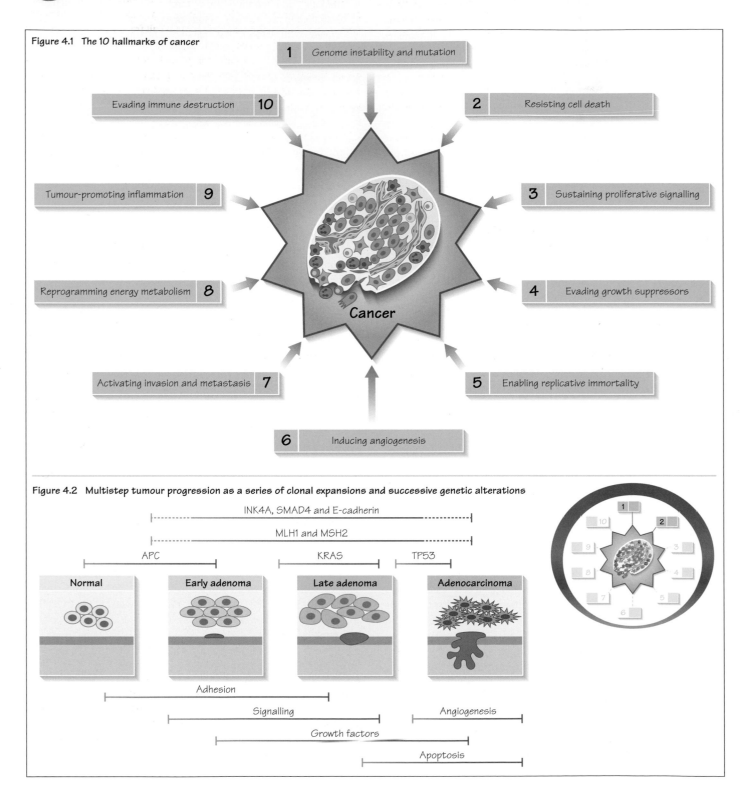

Figure 4.1 The 10 hallmarks of cancer

1 Genome instability and mutation

10 Evading immune destruction

2 Resisting cell death

9 Tumour-promoting inflammation

3 Sustaining proliferative signalling

8 Reprogramming energy metabolism

4 Evading growth suppressors

7 Activating invasion and metastasis

5 Enabling replicative immortality

6 Inducing angiogenesis

Cancer

Figure 4.2 Multistep tumour progression as a series of clonal expansions and successive genetic alterations

INK4A, SMAD4 and E-cadherin

MLH1 and MSH2

APC   KRAS   TP53

Normal   Early adenoma   Late adenoma   Adenocarcinoma

Adhesion

Signalling   Angiogenesis

Growth factors

Apoptosis

The 10 hallmarks of cancer (Figure 4.1)

It is likely that all multicellular organisms are affected, or have the potential to be affected, by cancer. Paleopathologists have demonstrated cancerous lesions in the long bones of dinosaurs long before the advent of *Homo sapiens*. The Edwin Smith papyrus includes a glyph clearly outlining a cancer of the breast, proving the Ancient Egyptians knew of the existence of cancer in humans.

There have been considerable advances in the knowledge and understanding of cancer since these early records. The formation and growth of cancer is a multistep process, during which sequentially occurring gene mutations result in the formation of a cancerous cell. For cells to be able to initiate carcinogenesis successfully, they need to acquire a set of key cellular characteristics. A number of these key features, collectively referred to as the hallmarks of cancer, are required for cancer cells to survive, proliferate and disseminate successfully, and these are discussed in the next four chapters.

1. Genome instability and mutation

Genomic instability is undoubtedly the most important factor for the development of the cancer cell. Random genetic mutations occur continuously throughout all cells of the body but these changes are rarely associated with significant phenotypic alterations. Occasionally, mutations confer a selective advantage to single cells, allowing overgrowth and dominance of these cells in local tissue environments. Multistep carcinogenesis occurs as a result of successive clonal expansions of premalignant cells, with each expansion being triggered by the acquisition of a random enabling genetic mutation.

Small alterations and mutations may happen continuously but cellular DNA repair mechanisms are so effective that almost all spontaneous mutations are corrected without ever producing phenotypic changes. Therefore, the overall mutation rates are kept very low. However, in cancer cells the accumulation of mutations can be accelerated by compromising the surveillance systems that normally monitor genomic integrity and force genetically damaged cells into either senescence or apoptosis. Therefore, they can become more sensitive to mutagenic actions or develop DNA repair mechanism failure.

2. Resisting cell death

There are three principal mechanisms through which cell death occurs in healthy tissues.

Apoptosis is programmed cell death and is frequently found to occur at markedly reduced rates in tumours, particularly those of high malignant grade or those resistant to treatment. The cellular apoptotic system is composed of upstream regulatory elements, which sense intrinsic and extrinsic proapoptotic signals, and downstream effector components, which are responsible for the execution of apoptosis.

In response to signalling from regulatory elements, effectors initiate a cascade of proteolysis and cell disassembly, resulting in a sequence of programmed cell death. This produces nuclear fragmentation, chromosomal condensation, shrinking of the cell with loss of intercellular contact followed by blebbing of the cell membrane, cellular fragmentation and the formation of apoptotic bodies that are subsequently phagocytosed by neighbouring cells.

Apoptosis can result from multiple stimuli or indeed from the removal of survival factors such as IL-3 or IGF-1.

Lack of survival factors is particularly important during development as this prevents cells migrating to wrong areas or structures. Direct signals to produce cell death can result from interaction between cytokines and cell surface receptors. Furthermore, if there is an imbalance between factors required for normal proliferation, such as when cyclin E is activated without cyclin D, it can result in apoptosis. This may appear confusing, as the same genes that are used for normal cell proliferation can also trigger apoptosis if they are inactivated inappropriately. However, the most important regulator of apoptosis is the *TP53* tumour suppressor gene. *TP53* is often described as the 'guardian of the genome' because it is able to induce apoptosis in response to sufficient levels of genomic damage. The largest initiator of apoptosis via *TP53* is cellular injury, particularly due to DNA damage resulting from chemotherapy, oxidative damage and UV radiation. When *TP53* tumour suppressor function is lost in cancerous cells, a central control element of apoptosis is disabled.

Cancer cells will most commonly demonstrate loss of *TP53* tumour suppressor function. Other triggers include increased expression of antiapoptotic regulators (Bcl-2, Bcl-xL) or survival signals, downregulation of proapoptotic factors (Bax, Bim, Puma) and short-circuiting of the extrinsic ligand-induced death pathway.

Autophagy is a catabolic process during which cellular constituents are degraded by lysosomal machinery within the cell. It is an important physiological mechanism, which usually occurs at low levels in cells but can be induced in response to environmental stresses, particularly in circumstances of nutrient deficiency. The cellular metabolites produced are recycled and used for biosynthetic and metabolic purposes by the cell, a mechanism that is particularly useful in the nutrient-poor environments encountered by expanding cancer cell populations.

Paradoxically, in addition to nutrient starvation, radiotherapy and cytotoxic chemotherapy induce elevated levels of autophagy that are cytoprotective for malignant cells, thus impeding rather than perpetuating the killing actions of these stress situations. Severely stressed cancer cells have been shown to shrink via autophagy to a state of reversible dormancy. This survival response may enable the persistence and eventual regrowth of some late-stage tumours following treatment with potent anticancer agents.

Necrosis is premature death of cells and is characterised by the release of cellular contents into the local tissue microenvironment. This stands in marked contrast to apoptosis, where cells are disassembled in a step-by-step fashion and the resulting cellular fragments are phagocytosed. Necrotic cell death results in the recruitment of inflammatory immune cells to the site of tissue damage.

There is strong evidence to suggest that these cells have tumour-promoting properties in the context of carcinogenesis, as they have been shown to promote angiogenesis, cellular proliferation and tissue invasion in experimental conditions. In addition, necrotic cells release stimulatory factors, which promote proliferation of neighbouring cells and potentially contribute to cancer development. As a consequence, necrotic cell death within cancer cell populations may promote rather than inhibit carcinogenesis.

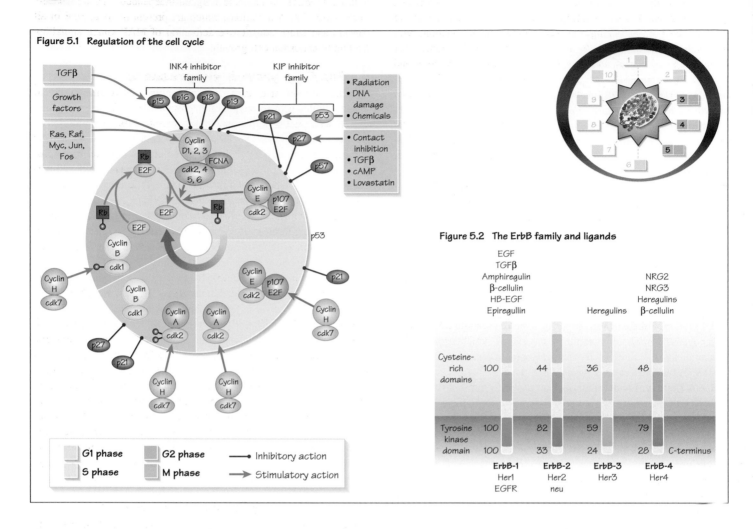

Figure 5.1 Regulation of the cell cycle

Figure 5.2 The ErbB family and ligands

3. Sustaining proliferative signalling

One of the most defining features of cancer cells is their ability to sustain proliferation beyond what would be expected for normal cells. Healthy tissues maintain homeostasis through strict regulation of growth-promoting signalling pathways, which are responsible for driving progression of cells through the cell cycle. These signalling mechanisms are deregulated in cancerous cells. Growth-promoting signalling pathways typically involve growth factors, which are able to bind to cell surface-bound growth factor receptors. Binding of the ligand to receptors activates an intracellular tyrosine kinase-mediated signalling cascade, which ultimately leads to changes in gene expression, promoting cellular proliferation and growth. There are several different ways in which cancer cells may acquire sustained proliferative capacity:

- overproduction of growth factor ligands;
- overproduction of growth factor receptors;
- production of structurally altered receptors, which are able to signal in absence of ligand binding;
- activation of intracellular signalling pathway components so that signalling is no longer ligand-dependent

The cell cycle

The cell cycle is comprised of four ordered, strictly regulated phases referred to as G_1 (gap 1), S (DNA synthesis), G_2 (gap 2) and M (mitosis/meiosis). Normal cells grown in culture will stop proliferating and enter a quiescent state called G_0 once they become confluent or are deprived of serum or growth factors. The first gap phase (G_1) prior to the initiation of DNA synthesis, represents the period of commitment that separates M and S phases as cells prepare for DNA duplication. Cells in G_0 and G_1 are receptive to growth signals but once they have passed a restriction point they are committed to enter DNA synthesis (S phase). Cells demonstrate arrest at different points in G_1 in response to different inhibitory growth signals. Mitogenic signals promote progression through G_1 to S phase utilising phosphorylation of the retinoblastoma gene product (pRb). Following DNA synthesis there is a second gap phase (G_2) prior to mitosis (M) allowing cells to repair errors that have occurred during DNA replication and thus preventing propagation of these errors to daughter cells. Although the duration of individual phases may vary, depending on cell and tissue type, most adult cells are in a G_0 state at any one time.

Cell cycle regulation

The cell cycle is orchestrated by a number of molecular mechanisms, most importantly the key regulatory elements known as cyclins and cyclin-dependent kinases (CDKs). Cyclins bind to CDKs, and are regulated by both activating and inactivating phosphorylation, with two main checkpoints at G_1/S and G_2/M transition. The genes that inhibit progression play an important part in tumour prevention and are thus referred to as tumour suppressor genes (e.g. *TP53*, *TP21*, *TP16* genes). The products of these genes deactivate the cyclin–CDK complexes and are thus able to halt the cell cycle.

The complexity of cell cycle control is susceptible to dysregulation, which may produce a malignant phenotype. This can result from loss of sensitivity to growth-inhibitory cytokines, loss of differentiation, loss of senescence, or from functional loss of the CDK inhibitors. A characteristic of the malignant phenotype is the lack of restriction prior to entry into S phase, so that cells with DNA damage do not arrest for repair, but instead duplicate the damaged genome and accumulate genetic changes that are likely to result in a proliferative advantage for the next generations.

Understanding the cell cycle has been essential for the development of many chemotherapy agents to target the cancer cells. Actively replicating cells are susceptible to damage by chemotherapy agents or radiation. Examples of this include antimetabolites that prevent purines and pyrimidines from becoming incorporated into DNA during S phase, and the mitotic spindle poisons, which inhibit assembly of tubulin into microtubules and thus disrupt the M phase by preventing the kinetochore separating the chromosomes. Some cytotoxics, on the other hand, such as the antibiotics and alkylating agents, affect the cell cycle in a non-specific way.

Stimulation of the cell cycle

Many cancer cells produce growth factors that drive their own proliferation by a positive feedback loop, a process known as autocrine stimulation. Examples include transforming growth factor alpha (TGF-α) and platelet-derived growth factor (PDGF). Progression through G_1 into S phase is regulated by cyclin D-, cyclin E- and cyclin A-associated kinases. D-type cyclins phosphorylate pRb and are responsible for progression through G_1 phase and re-entry into the cell cycle from G_0. E-type cyclins associate with CDK2 and stimulate transition through G_1 phase in combination with cyclin D and facilitates transition into S phase (see figure 5.1).

Other cancer cells express growth factor receptors at increased levels due to gene amplification or express abnormal receptors that are permanently activated. This results in abnormal cell growth in response to physiological growth factor stimulation or even in the absence of growth factor stimulation (ligand-independent signalling). The epidermal growth factor receptor (EGFR) is often over-expressed in lung and gastrointestinal tumours and the HER2 receptor is frequently over-expressed in breast cancer. Both receptors activate the Ras-Raf-MAP kinase pathway, causing cell proliferation, and understanding these effects has been vital for the development of novel therapies targeted to these receptors. An example of ligand-independent signalling occurs in the case of *RAS* mutations, which are present in about 30% of all cancers and cause constitutive activation of MAP kinase signalling leading to abnormal cell growth.

4. Evading growth suppressors

A further important characteristic of cancer cells is their ability to evade cellular growth suppression programmes, most of which are dependent on the action of tumour suppressor genes. The prototypical tumour suppressors *Rb* and *TP53* function as central control elements in cellular regulatory networks. They are able to halt cell cycle progression or induce cell death if excessive genome damage or suboptimal extracellular growth conditions occur. Cancer cells are able to proliferate independently of these inhibitory signals.

In healthy tissues, close cell-to-cell contact in dense cell populations also acts as an inhibitory factor on cell proliferation. This mechanism, known as contact inhibition, is typically absent in many cancer cell populations.

Growth-inhibitory factors can modulate the cell cycle regulators and produce activation of the CDK inhibitors, causing inhibition of the CDKs.

Mutations within inhibitory proteins are common in cancer. Loss of restriction by phosphorylated pRb can be found in human tumours, due to disruption of the pRb regulation pathway, which produces a loss of restraint on transition from G_1 to S phase of the cell cycle. Mutations in members of the *KIP* gene family are less common in human tumours; however, disruption of p53 function will have downstream effects on p21, which affects the coordination of DNA repair with cycle arrest, resulting in the affected cell accumulating genomic defects. Downregulation of p21 and p27, which can be found in tumours with normal p53 function, correlates notably with high tumour grade and poor prognosis.

5. Enabling replicative immortality

For cancer cells to be able to produce macroscopic tumours, they need to acquire the ability for unlimited proliferation. Telomeric DNA sequences, which protect and stabilise chromosomal ends, play a central role in conferring this limitless replicative potential. During replication of normal cells, telomeres shorten progressively as small fragments of telomeric DNA are lost with successive cycles of replication. This shortening process is thought to represent a mitotic clock and eventually prevents the cell from dividing further. Telomerase, a specialised polymerase enzyme, adds nucleotides to telomeres, allowing continued cell division and thus preventing premature arrest of cellular replication. The telomerase enzyme is almost absent in normal cells but expressed at significant levels in many human cancers.

6 The hallmarks of cancer III

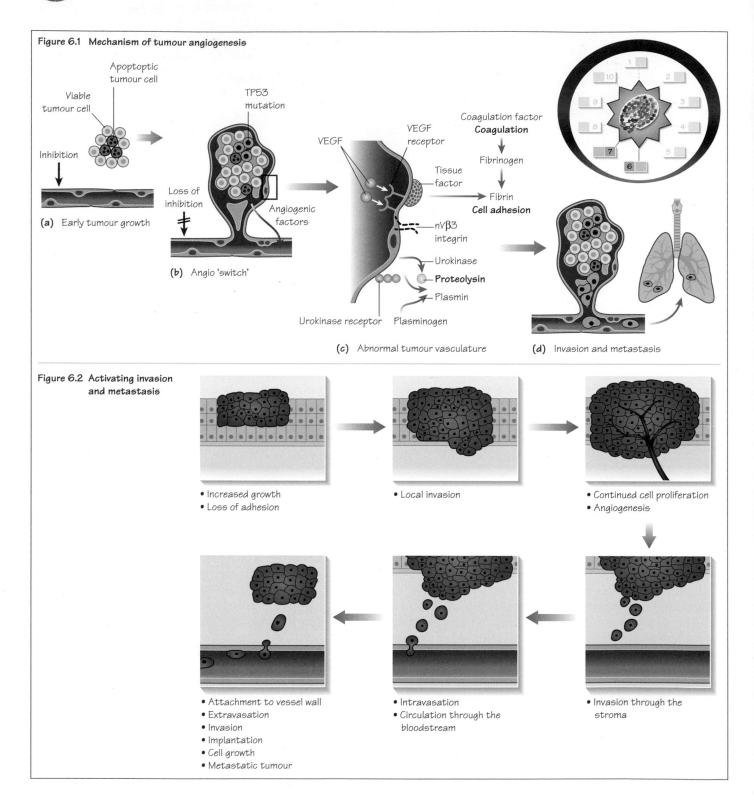

Figure 6.1 Mechanism of tumour angiogenesis

Viable tumour cell
Apoptoptic tumour cell
Inhibition
(a) Early tumour growth

TP53 mutation
Loss of inhibition
Angiogenic factors
(b) Angio 'switch'

VEGF
VEGF receptor
Tissue factor
nVβ3 integrin
Urokinase
Proteolysin
Plasmin
Urokinase receptor
Plasminogen
(c) Abnormal tumour vasculature

Coagulation factor
Coagulation
Fibrinogen
Fibrin
Cell adhesion

(d) Invasion and metastasis

Figure 6.2 Activating invasion and metastasis

- Increased growth
- Loss of adhesion

- Local invasion

- Continued cell proliferation
- Angiogenesis

- Invasion through the stroma

- Intravasation
- Circulation through the bloodstream

- Attachment to vessel wall
- Extravasation
- Invasion
- Implantation
- Cell growth
- Metastatic tumour

6. Inducing angiogenesis

All cancers require a functional vascular network to ensure continued growth and will be unable to grow beyond 1 mm³ without stimulating the development of a vascular supply. Tumours require sustenance in the form of nutrients and oxygen as well as an ability to evacuate metabolic waste products and carbon dioxide. This requires the development of new blood vessels, which is termed angiogenesis (Figure 6.1).

In an adult, the normal vasculature is largely quiescent, but as part of certain physiological processes, such as wound healing and female reproductive cycling, angiogenesis is transiently turned on. Blood vessels produced by tumour-mediated angiogenesis are abnormal and do not follow the normal patterns of vascular development. They are characterised by:

- precocious capillary sprouting;
- increased vessel branching;
- distorted and enlarged vessels;
- microhaemorrhage and leakiness;
- abnormal levels of endothelial cell proliferation and apoptosis.

Angiogenesis is dependent on the production of angiogenic growth factors, of which vascular endothelial growth factor (VEGF) and platelet-derived endothelial growth factor (PDGF) are the best characterised. During tumour progression, an angiogenic switch is activated and remains on, causing normally quiescent vasculature to continually sprout new vessels that help sustain expanding tumour growth. Angiogenesis is governed by a balance of proangiogenic stimuli and angiogenesis inhibitors, such as TSP-1, which binds to transmembrane receptors on endothelial cells and evokes suppressive signals.

A number of cells can contribute to the maintenance of a functional tumour vasculature and therefore sustain angiogenesis. These include pericytes and a variety of bone marrow-derived cells, such as; macrophages, neutrophils, mast cells and myeloid progenitors.

The requirement for cancer to promote angiogenesis has been exploited therapeutically in the development of agents that target angiogenic molecules or their receptors. Examples include bevacizumab (an antibody against VEGF) and sunitinib (a small molecule inhibitor of the PDGF receptor). Bevacizumab has been shown to improve survival for metastatic colon, breast and ovarian cancer; while sunitinib is useful in the treatment of renal cell cancer and as second-line treatment in gastrointestinal stromal tumours.

7. Activating invasion and metastasis

Invasion and metastasis are complex processes involving multiple discrete steps. They begin with local tissue invasion followed by infiltration of nearby blood and lymphatic vessels with cancerous cells. Malignant cells are eventually transported through haematogenous and lymphatic spread to distant sites within the body, where they form micrometastases, which will eventually grow into macroscopic metastatic lesions (Figure 6.2).

Cancer cells undergo a number of modifications as they progress through the different stages of invasion and metastasis. These alterations include changes in cell shape as well as changes in attachments to neighbouring cells and the surrounding extracellular matrix.

Cadherin-1 (epithelial- or E-cadherin) is a calcium-dependent cell-cell adhesion glycoprotein composed of five extracellular cadherin repeats, a transmembrane region and a highly conserved cytoplasmic tail. The ectodomain of this protein mediates bacterial adhesion to mammalian cells, and the cytoplasmic domain is required for internalisation. Cadherin-1 facilitates assembly of organised cell sheets in tissues. Increased expression of cadherin-1 is recognised as an antagonist of invasion and metastasis and in situ tumours usually retain cadherin-1 production.

Mutations in the encoding *CDH1* gene are associated with gastric, breast, colorectal, thyroid and ovarian cancers. Loss of cadherin-1 production due to downregulation or occasional mutational inactivation of *CDH1* has been observed in human cancers and this evidence supports the theory that *CDH1* plays a key role in suppression of invasion and metastasis.

Cadherin-1 downregulation decreases the strength of cellular adhesion within tissues, resulting in an increase in cellular motility. This in turn may allow cancer cells to cross the basement membrane and invade surrounding tissues. Expression of cadherin-1 is used by pathologists to differentiate between different forms of breast cancer. When compared with invasive duct carcinoma, cadherin-1 expression is markedly reduced or absent in the great majority of invasive lobular carcinomas when studied by immunohistochemistry.

The epithelial-mesenchymal transition results in the formation of new tumour colonies of cancer cells that exhibit features similar to those of primary tumour cells. The transformed epithelial cells may acquire the ability to invade, resist apoptosis and to disseminate. Cancer cells can concomitantly acquire multiple attributes that enable invasion and metastasis.

Crosstalk between cancer cells and cells of the surrounding stromal tissue is involved in the acquired capability for invasive growth and metastasis. Mesenchymal stem cells in tumour stroma have been found to secrete CCL5, a protein chemokine that helps recruit leukocytes into inflammatory sites. With the help of particular T-cell derived cytokines (IL-2 and IFN-γ), CCL5 induces proliferation and activation of natural killer cells and then acts reciprocally on cancer cells to stimulate invasive behaviour. Macrophages at the tumour periphery can foster local invasion by supplying matrix-degrading enzymes such as metalloproteinases and cysteine cathepsin proteases.

7 The hallmarks of cancer IV

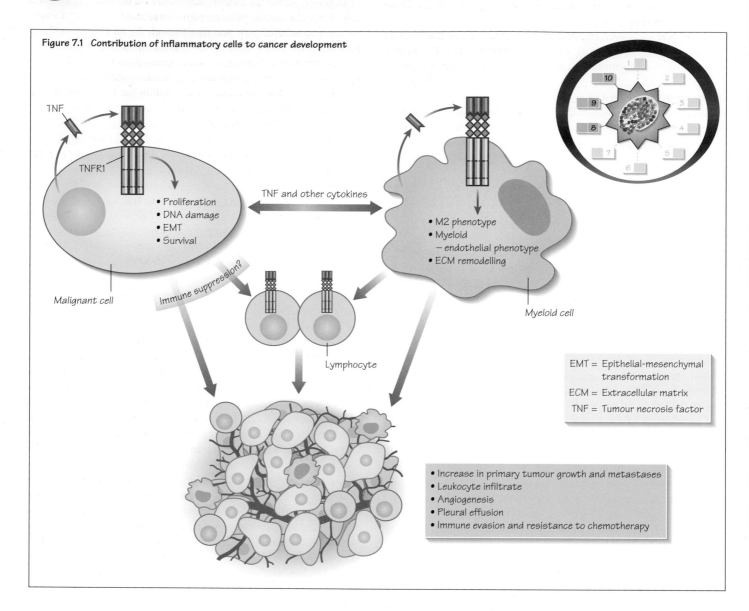

Figure 7.1 Contribution of inflammatory cells to cancer development

8. Reprogramming energy metabolism

Uncontrolled proliferation of malignant cells relies not only on loss of cell cycle control mechanisms but also requires adjustments of cellular energy metabolism.

Under aerobic conditions, oxidative phosphorylation functions as the main metabolic pathway for energy production; cells process glucose, first to pyruvate via glycolysis and thereafter to carbon dioxide in the mitochondria. Under anaerobic conditions, glycolysis is favoured to produce ATP.

Cancer cells can reprogram their glucose metabolism to limit energy production to glycolysis even in the presence of oxygen. This has been termed 'aerobic glycolysis'. Upregulation of glucose transporters such as GLUT1 is the main mechanism through which aerobic glycolysis is achieved.

This reprogramming of energy metabolism appears paradoxical, as overall energy production from glycolysis is significantly lower (18-fold) than that from oxidative phosphorylation. One explanation for this may be that amplification of glycolysis results in increased production of glycolytic intermediates. These metabolites may then be fed into various biosynthetic pathways, including those that generate the nucleosides and amino acids, which are necessary for the production of new cells. Some cancers have been found to contain two subpopulations of malignant cells that differ in their energy-generating pathways. One subpopulation consists of glucose-dependent cells that secrete lactate, whereas the second preferentially import and utilise the lactate produced by their neighbours as their main energy source, employing part of the citric acid cycle to do so.

9. Tumour-promoting inflammation

Almost all tumours show infiltration with immune cells on pathological investigation and historically this finding was thought to represent an attempt of the immune system to eradicate the cancer.

However, it is now clear that tumour-associated inflammatory responses promote tumour formation and cancer progression. Inflammatory vasodilation results in increased blood flow, while increased permeability of the blood vessels results in exudation (leakage) of plasma proteins and fluid into tissues, which manifests as swelling.

Cytokines are able to alter blood vessels to permit migration of leukocytes (mainly neutrophils), which permeate from the blood vessels into the tissue, a process known as extravasation. The inflammatory cytokines also promote immediate expression of P-selectin, or alternatively cadherin-1 on the surface of endothelial cells, which in turn bind weakly to carbohydrate ligands on the leukocytes, causing them to roll along the endothelial surface. Immunoglobulin ligands such as ICAM-1 and VCAM-1 are upregulated on endothelial cells, further slowing the migration of leukocytes. Leukocytes then become firmly bound to tumour-associated endothelial cells via integrin receptors for immunoglobulin ligands.

Migration across the endothelium occurs via the process of diapedesis, where chemokine gradients stimulate adhered leukocytes to move between endothelial cells and pass through the basement membrane into the surrounding tissues. The movement of leukocytes within tissues occurs via chemotaxis, where chemoattractants cause leukocytes to move along chemotactic gradients towards the source of chemokines within the tumour. Once within the tissue interstitium, leukocytes bind to extracellular matrix proteins via integrins and CD44 to prevent their loss from the site.

In addition to cell-derived mediators, several acellular biochemical cascade systems consisting of preformed plasma proteins act in parallel to initiate and propagate the inflammatory response. These include the complement system activated by bacteria, and the coagulation and fibrinolytic systems activated by necrosis, and they may occur in burns and trauma, as well as cancer. Other bioactive molecules such as growth factors and proangiogenic factors may be released by inflammatory immune cells into the surrounding tumour microenvironment. In particular, the release of reactive oxygen species, which are actively mutagenic, will accelerate the genetic evolution of surrounding cancer cells, enhancing growth and contributing to progression of the cancer.

10. Evading immune destruction

The immune system operates as a significant barrier to tumour formation and progression, and a hallmark of cancer development is the ability to escape from immunity. Cancer cells continuously shed surface antigens into the circulatory system, which prompts an immune response that includes cytotoxic T-cell, natural killer cell and macrophage production. It is thought that the immune system provides continuous surveillance, with resultant elimination of cells that undergo malignant transformation.

However, deficiencies in the development or function of CD8+ cytotoxic T lymphocytes, CD4+ Th1 helper T cells, or natural killer cells can each lead to a demonstrable increase in cancer incidence. Furthermore, highly immunogenic cancer cells may evade immune destruction by disabling components of the immune system. This is done through recruitment of inflammatory cells, including regulatory T cells and myeloid-derived suppressor cells, which are both actively immunosuppressive against the actions of cytotoxic lymphocytes (Figure 7.1).

Cancers will develop and progress when there is a loss of recognition by the immune system, a lack of susceptibility due to escape from immune cell action and induction of immune dysfunction, often via inflammatory mediators.

Table 8.1 Inherited cancer predisposition syndromes

Syndrome	Associated cancers	Inheritance	Gene
Ataxia telangiectasia	Leukaemia, lymphoma, ovary, gastric, brain, colon	AR	ATM
Breast–ovarian syndrome	Breast, ovary, colon, prostate, pancreas	AD	BRCA1, BRCA2
Bloom syndrome	Leukaemia, tongue, oesophagus, colon, Wilm's tumour	AR	BLM
Cowden syndrome	Breast, thyroid, gastrointestinal tract, pancreas	AD	PTEN
Familial adenomatous polyposis	Colon, upper gastrointestinal tract	AD	APC
Fanconi anaemia	Leukaemia, oesophagus, skin, hepatoma	AR	FACA, FACC, FACD
Gorlin syndrome	Basal cell skin, brain	AD	PTCH
Hereditary non-polyposis colon cancer	Colon, endometrium, ovary, pancreatic, gastric	AD	MSH2, MLH1, PMS1, PMS2
Li–Fraumeni syndrome	Sarcoma, breast, lung, colon, leukaemia, glioma, adrenocortical	AD	TP53
Melanoma	Melanoma	AD	CDK2 (p16)
MEN-1	Pancreatic islet cell, pituitary adenoma	AD	MEN1
MEN-2	Medullary thyroid carcinoma, phaeochromocytoma	AD	RET
Neurofibromatosis 1	Neurofibrosarcoma, phaeochromocytoma, optic glioma	AD	NF1
Neurofibromatosis 2	Vestibular schwannoma	AD	NF2
Papillary renal cell cancer syndrome	Renal cell cancer	AD	MET
Peutz–Jeghers syndrome	Colon, ileum, breast, ovary	AD	STK11
Prostate cancer	Prostate	AD	HPC1
Retinoblastoma	Retinoblastoma, osteosarcoma, small-cell lung cancer	AD	RB1
von Hippel–Lindau syndrome	Haemangioblastoma of retina and central nervous system, renal cell, phaeochromocytoma	AD	VHL
Wilm's tumour	Nephroblastoma, neuroblastoma, hepatoblastoma, rhabdomyosarcoma	AD	WT1
Xeroderma pigmentosa	Skin, leukaemia, melanoma	AR	XPA, XPC, XPD (ERCC2), XPF

AD = autosomal dominant, AR = autosomal recessive

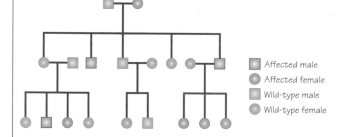

Figure 8.1 Autosominal dominant pedigree

Affected male
Affected female
Wild-type male
Wild-type female

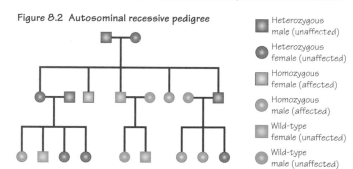

Figure 8.2 Autosominal recessive pedigree

Heterozygous male (unaffected)
Heterozygous female (unaffected)
Homozygous female (affected)
Homozygous male (affected)
Wild-type female (unaffected)
Wild-type male (unaffected)

Principles of cancer genetics

Cancer genetics encompasses two related but fundamentally different genetic concepts, the concept of germline mutation and that of somatic mutation.

Germline mutations are genetic changes in an individual's DNA that were present at embryogenesis. Consequently, these changes will affect all cells in that person's body, including germ cells and gametes, and can potentially be passed on to offspring. Germline mutations in cancer-causing genes are associated with hereditary cancer syndromes.

Somatic mutations are acquired genetic changes that occur within the DNA of individual somatic cells within the body. In contrast to germline mutations, somatic mutations only affect cells in which they originally occurred and direct descendants of these cells, and will not be detectable in unaffected tissues. The changes are non-inheritable as genetic alterations are not present in germ cells or gametes and so somatic mutations play an important role in the development of sporadic cancers.

What is potentially confusing is the fact that somatic mutations and germline mutations may potentially affect the same genes. For example, somatic mutations in the *APC* gene are frequently present in sporadic colorectal cancer, but mutations in the same gene are found in familial cases of colorectal cancer with inherited germline *APC* mutations (familial adenomatous polyposis).

While it is essential to identify the genes involved in hereditary cancer syndromes, it is useful to examine the genetic changes occurring in sporadic tumours. Identifying the mutations present results in increased understanding of the molecular biology of the cancer, allows classification of tumour subtypes and facilitates the development of targeted therapies. HER2 over-expression in breast cancers confers resistance to conventional treatment with taxane chemotherapy but indicates sensitivity to treatment with the monoclonal antibody trastuzumab (Herceptin), and HER2 testing is now a routine investigation in the clinic.

How genes cause cancer

A number of biological processes are well characterised in cancer cells, which typically:

- proliferate in the absence of growth factors;
- fail to respond to proliferation inhibition;
- evade apoptosis and senescence;
- recruit new blood vessels to enhance growth;
- invade surrounding tissues and metastasise.

Cell growth and proliferation are under tight genetic control in normal cells and healthy tissues, and loss of this control may result in the development of cancer. Oncogenes and tumour suppressor genes are classes of genes in which mutations are known to cause cancer.

Oncogenes

Oncogenes are mutated proto-oncogenes, which function in normal cells to promote cellular proliferation. They mostly encode growth factors, growth factor receptors, signal transducers, or transcription factors, and when mutated may become inappropriately active or insensitive to inactivating signals. Oncogenic changes are a 'gain of function' mutation and due to their activating nature only one gene copy needs to be affected for uncontrolled cell growth to occur. As a result, oncogenic mutations behave in a dominant manner at a cellular level.

Tumour suppressor genes

When working correctly, tumour suppressor genes function to inhibit cell proliferation. They can be genes involved in cell cycle control, DNA repair, apoptosis promotion, or telomerase regulation. Mutations in tumour suppressor genes are 'loss of function' mutations and both gene copies need to be rendered ineffective for changes in cellular function to occur. For this reason, tumour suppressor gene mutations are described as being recessive at a cellular level. In sporadic cancers this means that both functional gene copies have to be lost by mutation within the same cell. In the case of inherited cancers, one defective copy is inherited as a germline mutation and is thus present in all cells ('first hit'). The second gene copy becomes ineffective through somatic mutation usually only in a single cell or a small number of cells ('second hit'). This phenomenon was first described as the two hit hypothesis by Alfred Knudson in 1971.

One confusing aspect about tumour suppressor gene-associated inherited cancers is the fact that they can sometimes follow dominant inheritance patterns despite mutations being recessive at a cellular level. The two hit hypothesis can help explain this paradox as it is believed that inheritance of one defective tumour suppressor allele is insufficient to cause disease on its own, but is associated with a high rate of somatic mutation at the second gene copy which accounts for the dominant inheritance pattern.

Multistep carcinogenesis

The vast majority of human cancers (90%) are not familial or the consequence of known hereditary mutations. Nevertheless, many sporadic tumours are characterised by the presence of multiple sequential somatic gene changes which precede cancer development, and this process is known as multistep carcinogenesis. This phenomenon occurs in many tumour types but has been particularly well characterised for colorectal cancer in which mutations in the *APC* gene result in the development of benign polyps with hyperplasia and progress through adenoma into carcinoma if further mutations occur in DNA mismatch repair genes.

Inherited cancer syndromes

Some cancers present as clusters in families and are collectively known as familial cancer, but hereditary cancers are those familial cancers for which a specific inheritance pattern has been identified (see Table 8.1). A detailed family history is essential to identify patients affected by the abnormal gene and those at risk of the cancer. Individuals with a suspected genetic predisposition should be referred to a cancer genetics service for counselling and appropriate risk assessment.

Autosomal dominant cancer syndromes

Some inherited cancer syndromes follow an autosomal dominant inheritance pattern, with each offspring having a 50% risk of inheriting the disease trait. Whether or not a carrier develops a cancer depends on the penetrance of the gene in question, which in turn is dependent on factors such as normal function of the mutated gene and the extent to which the functionality of the gene protein product is compromised by mutation. If penetrance of the mutated allele is high, up to 50% of the offspring may exhibit the cancer phenotype. Lynch syndrome is a well-known example of an autosomal dominant cancer syndrome, caused by inherited defects in one of several DNA mismatch repair genes. It is characterised by a significantly increased lifetime risk of developing colorectal, gastric, endometrial and ovarian cancer.

Autosomal recessive cancer syndromes

In autosomal recessive syndromes the cancer trait will only manifest if both maternal and paternal alleles of the gene in question carry the predisposition mutation. The probability of transmission to each offspring is only 25% if both parents are unaffected carriers of the mutated allele. Detecting recessive disorders can be challenging in clinical practice, particularly in families with small numbers of offspring per generation. An example of an autosomal recessive cancer syndrome is ataxia telangiectasia, which is caused by mutations in the *ATM* gene. This encodes a kinase protein essential for activity of the p53 protein. Ataxia telangiectasia is associated with an increased risk of haematological malignancies and breast cancer.

9 Communicating with cancer patients

Table 9.1 Outline of communication skill attributes

Communication skill	Definition	Example
Sign posting	Setting out objectives and a plan for the conversation to prepare both participants for what will and will not be covered. Outlining expectations	'The purpose of meeting today is…'
Active listening	Allow the other person to do the talking while you listen and make encouraging statements to facilitate further conversation	At the beginning of a consultation ask an open question and give the patient at least one minute to talk. Nod your head and usephrases such as 'uh- huh' and 'I see' to encourage them to continue
Reflecting	Repeating the patient's own words and phrases back to them to encourage clarification and elaboration	If the patient said 'I have been feeling different', just repeat the word 'different' and wait. This should prompt them to elaborate
Non-verbal cues and body language	The use of body positioning, voice tone and speed, etc., to convey information that may not be communicated verbally	Patients may be sitting with their arms folded or eyes to the floor showing they are uncomfortable with the topic or situation
Internal summary and final summary	Picking out the important points that have been covered and reiterating them. Internal summaries can be done at any point during the consultation based on points covered so far, whereas a summary is used at the very end	'So before we move on to talk about treatment, I would like to summarise what we have covered so far…'
Use of resources	Using other media to convey the messages of the conversation	The use of leaflets, support groups and websites give the patient time to digest information at their own pace
Empathy	The ability to understand another person's situation, perspective and feelings, and to communicate that understanding to them	Use phrases such as 'that must be veryhard for you', 'I see how that must be difficult'. Be careful not to over-empathise or pretend, as this could appear patronising

Table 9.2 Overcoming barriers to communication

Barrier to communication	Approach to good practice
Time management	Ensure that adequate time is available to cover both your own and the patient's agenda
Language and understanding	Avoid medical jargon or explain it immediately after use. If English is not a first language, then use interpreters or the telephone language service
Personal attitudes	Remain professional at all times and do not allow personal beliefs to influence the approach to communication
Preparation	Do not initiate a conversation or explanation unprepared, and ensure you have the required information available before explaining to a patient
Personal failings	Avoid consultations when you are excessively tired. It does not create a good impression and can result in poor communication
Environment	Ensure privacy for the conversation, with minimal background noise. Check that the patient is comfortable and has appropriate support available

Communicating with cancer patients

As in all specialities, good communication with patients is vital, but the emotional nature of cancer creates a potential barrier for both students and doctors in training. Furthermore, poor communication can result in medical, legal and ethical problems, precipitating strain on the patients and healthcare professionals.

Although healthcare professionals will have individual techniques for communicating with patients depending on their personality, most will follow some basic techniques. The key point is to understand what works best for you and to incorporate appropriate tools and tactics (Tables 9.1 and 9.2), while remembering that nothing is more transparent to a patient than speaking to someone who is 'acting'. It is important to develop insight into what may be preventing the patient from communicating effectively with you and vice versa. An awareness of any barriers to mutual communication is a key skill for the healthcare professional.

The doctor–patient relationship

Cancer patients are seen over long periods of time and often when emotions are at their most fraught. It is essential to create a trusting environment where the patient feels safe, and to establish expectations and professional boundaries at the primary consultation.

Patients should be involved in the planning of their own treatment and the role of an oncologist is to outline the diagnosis, implications, potential outcome and the rationale and expectations of treatment. Patients should be able to make informed decisions about their treatment or, indeed, the withdrawal of their treatment and planning of end of life care. Patients can feel overwhelmed with the treatment options available to them and clarity of communication is vital.

Breaking bad news

In order to break bad news, it is important to consider what this encompasses. 'Bad news' can be anything that negatively alters the patient's view of their future, resulting in a cognitive, behavioural, or emotional deficit in that person. It is important not to become so detached that one cannot realise that a patient is experiencing what may be bad news for them when you had not imagined it to be so. Every healthcare professional should be able to pre-empt a situation where bad news is to be shared and there are steps to follow that will help.

What is devastating to one person may be interpreted differently by another, emphasising the importance of using a patient-centred approach to the individual. Practising steps involved in breaking bad news can help doctors feel more comfortable when exposed to more challenging situations. When bad news is delivered poorly, the experience may stay in the mind of a patient or carer long after the initial shock of the news has been dealt with.

It is important not to forget that breaking bad news may be distressing for doctors as well, and to accept that an inability to cure does not signify failure. All healthcare professionals must ensure that they discuss any stress relating to these situations with suitable colleagues, allowing them to deal with any personal feelings and learn from others.

Steps to breaking bad news

Preparing for the consultation. Doctors should allow adequate time, select an appropriate environment and ensure that all the facts are correct. The patient may want a family member present. It is important to be on the same level as the patient rather than towering over them.

Setting the scene. Establishing what the patient already knows is essential, and reasons for the consultation should be made clear. It is also important to explore how much the patient wants to know. Some patients prefer to know very little about their condition, whereas others will ask very specific questions.

Warning shot. It may be appropriate to warn the patient that they are about to receive bad news. Statements such as: *'I am sorry to say that I have some bad news for you'* may allow patients to prepare for the news to come.

Chunking and checking. Patients should not be overloaded with information. Providing information in a step-by-step manner and checking that the information provided has been understood before proceeding will ensure that the patient understands what they are being told. Always encourage the patient to summarise the information provided, as this aids understanding.

Encouraging questions. Patients may wish to write down questions prior to consultations. Questions should always be answered honestly and, if this is not possible, doctors should admit this and make every effort to obtain the information requested by the patient. It can be useful to pre-empt questions one may be faced with.

Allowing the patient to express their emotions. The power of silence in facilitating this should not be underestimated.

Concerns and expectations. The patient's concerns and expectations should be explored, and it may be appropriate to speak to family members or carers.

Safety netting. Following the consultation, it may be useful to arrange a further appointment so that the patient has the opportunity to ask further questions having had time to process the information provided.

Providing leaflets. Leaflets and other resources may be provided where appropriate.

Documenting the consultation. Conversations should always be recorded in the patient's medical notes, including details of what was said, who was present and what further action was agreed. Accurate documentation will aid future consultations, and is vital from a legal viewpoint.

Dealing with the emotional patient

When a patient becomes emotional it is important that you react appropriately. As experience grows, you will feel more comfortable in dealing with such situations. Keeping calm and modelling this to the patient rather than asking the patient to calm down is essential. It is important to prepare for the unexpected, as each patient may react differently to others. Allowing time through pauses in the discussion gives the patient opportunity the to vent their feelings. Empathy rather than sympathy should be demonstrated at all times.

Communicating with younger patients

Cancer frequently affects children or young adults and communication may need to be adapted when dealing with this patient group. It is important to address both the patient and their parents or guardians, remembering that everyone should be involved in the discussions. It may be appropriate to speak to younger patients alone as they may not be open while there are others in the room. They may see doctors as an authority figure and it may take time for them to trust you before they open up and engage with you. Consider that maturity level may not always correlate with age; it is important to ensure that everyone understands the information you are discussing. Never patronise or oversimplify.

Some issues will have greater impact in younger patients. For example, hair loss from chemotherapy may have a more significant impact on a 19-year-old girl than the diagnosis of cancer. Younger patients often have a strong desire to fit in with their peers and it is vital that patients are able to share these concerns with their doctor.

It is best not to change your persona in an attempt to appear 'cool' in the false belief that this will make it easier for younger patients to relate to you. Usually, it will act as a barrier to communication and, if anything, will fuel mistrust. Be yourself and the patients will respect you and value their relationship with you and the care they receive.

Figure 10.1   Clinical examination of a patient suspected of having cancer

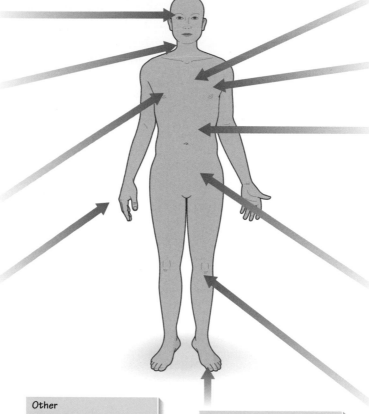

Face
- Conjunctival pallor
- Icterus, jaundice
- Horner's syndrome
- Cushingoid features
- Heliotrope rash

Lymph nodes
- Neck
- Supraclavicular
- Axillary
- Antecubital
- Inguinal
- Femoral
- Para-aortic

Breast examination
- Peau d'orange
- Puckering
- Erythema
- Nipple changes

Hands
- Clubbing
- HPOA
- Signs of smoking
- Pallor
- Tyelosis of palms

Observation
- Skin changes
- Ascites
- Cushingoid appearance
- Cachexia
- Dehydration
- Temperature (Pel–Ebstein)

Other
- Haematuria
- PV examination
- PR examination
- Fundoscopy

Periphery
- Calf tenderness (DVT)
- Clubbing (if present in hands)
- Ankle tenderness (HOA)

Cardiovascular
- SVC obstruction
- Atrial fibrillation
- Pericardial effusion
- Hypo-, hypertension

Respiratory
- Stridor, obstruction
- Consolidation
- Pleural effusion

Abdomen
- Surgical scars
- Umbilical nodule
- Mass in epigastrium
- Visible peristalsis
- Abdominal distension
- Ascites
- Hepatomegaly
- Splenomegaly
- Renal mass
- Pelvic mass
- Adenexal mass

Neurological
- Focal neurological signs
- Sensory deficit
- Spinal cord compression
- Memory deficit
- Personality change
- Cerebellar signs
- Myaesthenia gravis

Skeletal survey
- Focal bone tenderness (pelvis, spine, long bones)
- Wrist tenderness (HOA)

Table 10.1   Local features of malignant disease

Symptoms	Typical tumour primary site
Abdominal swelling (ascites)	Ovary, stomach, pancreas
Airway obstruction, stridor, cough, recurrent infection	Bronchus, thyroid
Bone pain or fracture	Bone (primary sarcoma, secondary metastasis from breast, prostate, bronchus, thyroid, kidney)
Change in bowel habit, abdominal discomfort or pain	Colon, rectum, ovary
Dysphagia	Oesophagus, bronchus, stomach
Haemorrhage	Stomach, colon, bronchus, endometrium, bladder, kidney
Jaundice	Hepatocellular carcinoma, lung, breast, colon, melanoma, stomach, oesophagus, endometrium, prostate, cervix, neuroendocrine tumours, renal
Lump	Breast, lymph node (any site), testis
Odynophagia, early satiety, vomiting	Bronchus, oesophagus, stomach, colon, rectum, ovary
Skin abnormality	Melanoma, basal cell carcinoma, all forms of skin cancer
Ulcer	Oesophagus, stomach, anus, skin

Presenting features of cancer

In the early stages of cancer development, the number of malignant cells is small and the patient is usually asymptomatic. With tumour progression, localised signs or symptoms develop due to mass effects and/or invasion of local tissues (Table 10.1). With further progression, symptoms may occur at distant sites as a result of metastatic disease or from non-metastatic manifestations due to the production of biologically active hormones by the tumour, or as the result of an immune response to antigens present on the tumour cells. Common presenting features are discussed below, with a suggested approach to examination of a patient suspected of having cancer.

General features on examination

Unintentional weight loss is a characteristic feature of advanced cancer, but can be due to other causes such as thyrotoxicosis, chronic inflammatory disease and chronic infective disorders. Fever can occur in any cancer secondary to infection, but may be a primary feature in Hodgkin's disease, lymphoma, leukaemia, renal cancer and liver cancer. The presence of unexplained weight loss or fever warrants investigation to exclude the presence of an occult malignancy. Weight gain is seen in patients with ascites or Cushing's syndrome (see Chapter 11). Patients with significant blood loss may demonstrate pallor due to anaemia, possibly from a primary site in the gastrointestinal or female genital tract.

Finger clubbing is a feature of many cancers, especially non-small cell lung cancer, although benign causes are recognised. Finger clubbing can be a feature of hypertrophic osteoarthropathy (HOA) in which there is periosteal new bone formation at the wrist and ankle (particularly seen in squamous cell lung cancer; see Chapter 30).

Local effects

A palpable mass or lump detected by the patient or physician may be the first sign of cancer. Primary tumours of the thyroid, breast, testis and skin are often detected in this way, whereas palpable lymph nodes in the neck, groin, or axilla may indicate secondary spread of tumour. A mass may produce pain or discomfort, which alerts the patient and clinician to a problem.

Lymph node examination of all regions is required as cancer will spread via the lymphatic system. It is particularly important when there is a presenting mass, where locoregional lymph nodes must be examined. Supraclavicular and axillary nodes are seen in cancer of the breast, lung, oesophagus and stomach, whereas nodes in the inguinal or femoral areas are more associated with cancers of the vagina, vulva, cervix and uterus.

Bleeding can result from a malignant lesion on a mucosal surface such as the stomach, bowel, bladder, bronchus, endometrium or kidney and can cause microscopic or macroscopic haemorrhage, in some cases producing significant blood loss and iron deficiency.

Skin abnormalities such as a change in pigmentation, size or characteristics of a skin lesion should be investigated. Skin changes can manifest due to an underlying malignancy as a non-metastatic effect (see Chapter 11).

Change of function

Dysphagia can result from oesophagogastric cancer or occasionally lung cancer. Characteristically, the symptoms are progressive and worse for solids than liquids. A local lesion in the large or small bowel can produce a change in bowel habit, ranging from diarrhoea to constipation. Constipation can result in bowel obstruction, producing nausea, vomiting and abdominal pain. Ovarian cancer can cause extrinsic compression of the bowel and present in a similar manner. Airway obstruction, recurrent chest infections, cough or stridor can result from lung cancer or occasionally from extrinsic compression as a result of enlargement of the thyroid. Early satiety (feeling full after small volumes of food) is a feature of liver metastasis (often due to cancer of the bronchus, stomach, oesophagus, colon, or rectum) but can be due to ascites alone.

Obstruction of a conduit

Obstruction of a body structure that acts as a conduit can produce jaundice (biliary tract in cholangiocarcinoma, pancreatic cancer), hydronephrosis (ureter in cervical cancer), bowel obstruction (colorectal cancer), bronchial obstruction (lung cancer), urethra restriction of urine flow (prostate cancer), lymphoedema of the arms or legs (lymph node infiltration).

Metastatic effects

Jaundice. The presence of jaundice suggests post-hepatic obstruction of the biliary tree or intrahepatic metastasis. Pre-hepatic jaundice due to autoimmune haemolysis is a rare feature of lymphoma. Obstructive jaundice is a more common feature of pancreatic, gastric and colorectal cancers, in addition to cholangiocarcinoma.

Breast examination. In a female patient presenting with widespread metastatic disease, bone pain or focal consolidation in the chest, examination of the breasts is required to explore a possible primary site. Normal breast examination does not exclude the diagnosis.

Bone pain or fracture. The presence of focal tenderness in the axial or peripheral skeleton should be investigated as metastasis can cause discomfort and functional impairment. Common cancers that involve bone include: breast, lung, thyroid, prostate and renal cancers. Primary cancers of bone such as osteosarcoma can present with a pathological fracture or pain and can be misdiagnosed as osteomyelitis.

Ascites or effusions. The production of an exudate will cause ascites in ovarian, pancreatic and gastric cancers. Pleural effusions can be seen in most cancers that have metastasised to the lungs or pleura but are particularly common in cancers of the ovary, breast, lung, pleura and stomach.

Organomegaly. The metastasis to an organ may produce enlargement (hepatomegaly or splenomegaly) or a change in texture found on palpation (firm, knobbly hepatomegaly in carcinoid syndrome). Hepatosplenomegaly with lymphadenopathy suggests a lymphoproliferative condition such as lymphoma.

Non-metastatic manifestations of cancer. These are considered separately (see Chapter 11).

11 Paraneoplastic syndromes

Table 11.1 Ectopic hormone production by tumours

Hormone	Consequence	Associated tumours
ACTH	Cushing's syndrome	SCLC
Activated factor X	Prothrombotic tendency (Trousseau syndrome)	Ovary, pancreas, breast, prostate
ADH	Hyponatraemia, confusion	SCLC, lymphoma, NSCLC (rarely)
Cytokines	Weight loss and anorexia	NSCLC, colorectal
Erythropoietin	Polycythaemia	Kidney, hepatoma, cerebellar haemangioblastoma, uterine fibroids (benign)
FGF23	Hypophosphataemic osteomalacia	Mesenchymal tumours
Gastrin	Peptic ulceration	Gastrinoma (Zollinger–Ellison syndrome)
Glucagon	Migratory necrolytic erythema, muscle wasting	Glucagonoma
β-hCG	Gynaecomastia	Germ cell tumours
Insulin	Hypoglycaemia	Insulinomas, mesenchymal tumours (also in advanced cancers)
Norepinephrine, epinephrine, dopamine	Hypertension, flushing, headache, palpitations	Phaeochromocytoma
Oestrogens	Gynaecomastia	Sertoli–Leydig cancer of the ovary or testis, hepatoma
PTHrP	Hypercalcaemia	NSCLC (squamous cell), breast, kidney, myeloma
Serotonin	Carcinoid syndrome	Neuroendocrine or carcinoid tumours
VIP	Watery diarrhoea, hypokalaemia	VIPoma (Werner–Morrison syndrome)

Cancer can manifest as signs and symptoms that may not be directly related to the cancer itself. These are known collectively as paraneoplastic syndromes and they exert a wide range of effects via depletion of normal factors, production of ectopic substances, or a host immunological response to the tumour.

Ectopic hormone production

In some cases, the first presentation of cancer is with a metabolic abnormality due to ectopic production of hormones by tumour cells, including insulin, ACTH, ADH, FGF23, erythropoietin, PTHrP and gonadotrophins (Table 11.1). If the cancer is successfully treated, the ectopic production is stopped and the metabolic abnormality resolves.

Cushing's syndrome can result from a pituitary adenoma (Cushing's disease), exogenous steroids, or an adrenal adenoma, but 20% of cases result from ectopic ACTH production. Patients can often present with the clinical features of hypercortisolism and hypokalaemic metabolic alkalosis with muscle weakness, hypertension, oedema, confusion, glucose intolerance and weight gain. Diagnosis can be confirmed by demonstrating a high 24-hour urinary free cortisol, high serum ACTH (>200 pg/mL) and failure to suppress ACTH production following a high-dose dexamethasone suppression test. Most cases (>50%) are associated with small cell lung cancer and neuroendocrine tumours (15%), such as phaeochromocytoma, carcinoid tumours, neuroblastoma and medullary cell carcinoma of the thyroid.

Carcinoid syndrome results from the production of serotonin, typically from the enterochromaffin cells in the gastrointestinal tract, pancreas and lungs. The serotonin and kinins are normally secreted into the portal circulation and undergo first-pass metabolism in the liver, and therefore none reaches the systemic circulation to cause symptoms. However, if the primary site is outside the portal circulation, or the patient has developed metastasis to the liver, then the release will be directly into the systemic circulation. This produces symptoms of vasomotor flushing, diarrhoea, wheezing, fever and abdominal pain. Chronic complications include tricuspid incompetence, cirrhosis, arthropathy and pellagra due to tryptophan deficiency. Diagnosis is by collection of 24-hour urine samples for 5-hydroxyindoleacetic acid (5-HIAA), which is a metabolite of 5-HT.

Neurological manifestations

These are a group of conditions associated with cancer that are thought to be due to an immunological response to antigens on the tumour cells, where the resulting antibodies cross-react with neurological or muscle tissue. These manifestations are rare but well characterised and can be the presenting feature in some patients, before the cancer is diagnosed. Furthermore, metastatic disease requires exclusion. The cancers most commonly implicated are those of the lung (small cell and non-small cell), pancreas, breast, prostate, ovary and lymphoma. Peripheral neuropathy can occur and is the result of axonal degeneration or demyelination. Encephalomyelitis can occur, especially in patients with small cell lung cancer, and can present with diverse symptoms depending on which region of the brain is involved. Cerebellar degeneration may be quite debilitating and usually presents with rapid onset of cerebellar ataxia, nystagmus and dysarthria. Lambert–Eaton myasthenic syndrome (LEMS) is due to an underlying cancer in about 60% of cases and is caused by the development of antibodies to presynaptic calcium channels. It presents with proximal muscle weakness, which improves on exercise. New onset of myasthenia-like ptosis should prompt consideration of an underlying malignancy.

When the manifestation is due to an autoimmune reaction to the tumour antigens, successful treatment of the cancer may remove the antigen but the autoantibodies of the immunological response are often unaffected. Therefore, the paraneoplastic effects can continue and be quite debilitating, despite successful treatment of the cancer.

Cutaneous manifestations

Many cancers can present with skin manifestations which are not due to metastases. Pruritis may be a presenting feature of lymphoma, leukaemia and CNS tumours. Acanthosis nigricans, characteristic thickening and darkening of skin in body folds and creases, may precede cancers by many years and is particularly associated with oesophagogastric cancer. Pemphigus may occur in lymphoma, Kaposi's sarcoma and thymic tumours. Vitiligo is associated with malignant melanoma, possibly mediated by an immune response to melanocytes.

Dermatomyositis is associated with an underlying malignancy in 40% of cases, such that patients require investigation for cancer. It is most commonly associated with oesophagogastric, lung, colorectal, ovarian and breast cancer. The juvenile form has a much lower association with cancer.

Erythema gyratum, with an appearance similar to wood grain, is strongly suggestive of an underlying malignancy (lung, breast, cervix, gastrointestinal). Almost half the patients with extramammary Paget's disease, often found in the genital and anal regions, have an underlying malignancy, most commonly in the breast, uterus, rectum, bladder, vagina, or prostate. Some cutaneous manifestations are secondary to ectopic hormones, including hirsutism and the cutaneous signs of Cushing's syndrome.

Haematological manifestations

This encompasses a wide range of abnormalities seen on full blood counts which may or may not cause symptoms. The most common abnormality is anaemia, typically a normocytic, normochromic anaemia of chronic disease. Hypochromic, microcytic iron deficiency anaemia can result from chronic blood loss in bowel cancers, and haemolytic anaemia is associated with leukaemia. Leukocytosis can result from the release of cytokines, seen particularly in lymphomas, gastric, lung, pancreatic and brain cancers. Eosinophilia is associated with Hodgkin's disease and mycosis fungoides. Leukocytopenia and pancytopenia are rarely paraneoplastic phenomena and much more likely to be due to anticancer treatments.

Cancer patients will often have a prothrombotic tendency known as Trousseau's syndrome, manifesting as deep vein thrombosis or pulmonary embolism, occasionally despite adequate anticoagulation. The highest risk is associated with adenocarcinoma, particularly of the pancreas, ovary, breast and prostate.

Gastrointestinal manifestations

Weight loss, anorexia and nausea are common in patients with cancer. They form the most prevalent paraneoplastic phenomenon of cancer anorexia and cachexia syndrome (CACS). Over half of patients with solid organ malignancy will have weight loss. A loss above 10% of total body weight is associated with a worse outcome. The cause is multifactorial, but is primarily due to pro-inflammatory cytokines released by the host in response to the tumour. This is exacerbated by an increase in basal metabolic requirement due to tumour bulk and by chemotherapy-induced nausea or cancer affecting the bowel either by obstruction or following surgical resection. Serum albumin levels are a poor indicator of the extent of CACS and treatment is by nutritional support. Steroids have been shown to stimulate appetite but are best used for a short course to minimise the risk of proximal muscle weakness. Cancers that affect the bowel can result in increased mucosal permeability, ulceration or lymphatic obstruction, which can all result in a protein-losing enteropathy producing a diminished nutritional hypoproteinaemic state resulting in ascites and peripheral oedema.

Renal manifestations

Immune complex deposition may cause glomerular problems. It is estimated that around 10% of patients with idiopathic nephrotic syndrome have an underlying cancer, most commonly in cancers of the stomach, lung and liver. Lymphoma, haematological malignancies and solid organ tumours can all produce various nephropathies.

Other paraneoplastic syndromes

Hypertrophic osteoarthopathy (HOA) is the combination of clubbing and periostosis, typically producing discomfort at the wrist and ankle. This is well recognised as a feature of squamous cell lung cancer but is also seen in lung metastases, bowel and oesophageal cancer.

Fever is a non-specific symptom of cancer and approximately 30% of cancer patients will develop fever at some point in their illness, as a result of cytokine release from the tumour. This is seen most commonly with leukaemia. It is important to exclude sepsis in unexplained fever in a cancer patient, particularly in those receiving myelosuppressive chemotherapy and in those who are neutropenic. Some fever patterns are characteristic for certain malignancies, such as the Pel–Ebstein fevers at night time in Hodgkin's disease.

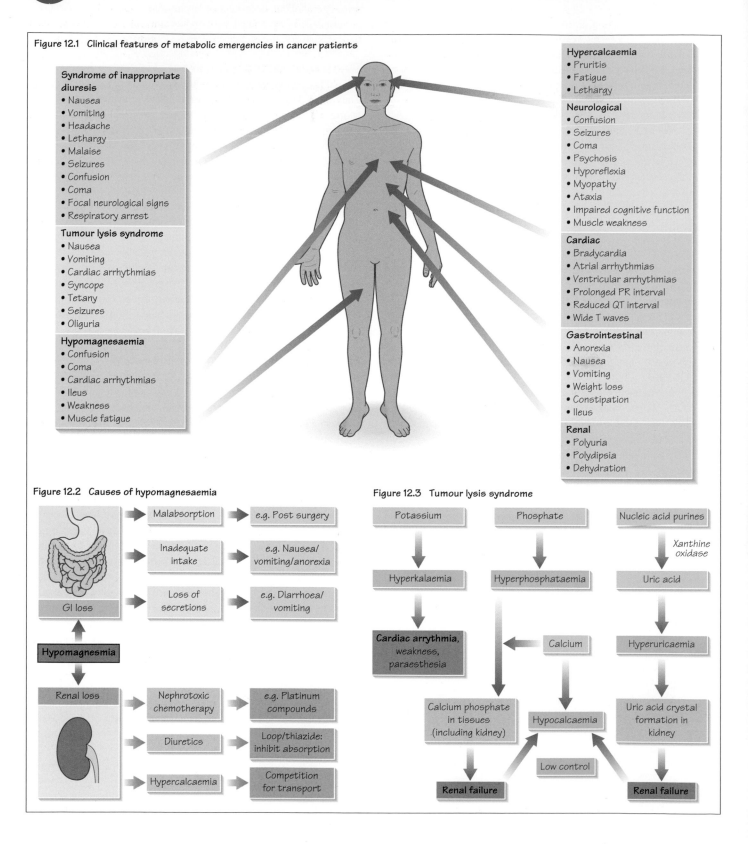

Figure 12.1 Clinical features of metabolic emergencies in cancer patients

Syndrome of inappropriate diuresis
- Nausea
- Vomiting
- Headache
- Lethargy
- Malaise
- Seizures
- Confusion
- Coma
- Focal neurological signs
- Respiratory arrest

Tumour lysis syndrome
- Nausea
- Vomiting
- Cardiac arrhythmias
- Syncope
- Tetany
- Seizures
- Oliguria

Hypomagnesaemia
- Confusion
- Coma
- Cardiac arrhythmias
- Ileus
- Weakness
- Muscle fatigue

Hypercalcaemia
- Pruritis
- Fatigue
- Lethargy

Neurological
- Confusion
- Seizures
- Coma
- Psychosis
- Hyporeflexia
- Myopathy
- Ataxia
- Impaired cognitive function
- Muscle weakness

Cardiac
- Bradycardia
- Atrial arrhythmias
- Ventricular arrhythmias
- Prolonged PR interval
- Reduced QT interval
- Wide T waves

Gastrointestinal
- Anorexia
- Nausea
- Vomiting
- Weight loss
- Constipation
- Ileus

Renal
- Polyuria
- Polydipsia
- Dehydration

Figure 12.2 Causes of hypomagnesaemia

GI loss → Malabsorption → e.g. Post surgery
GI loss → Inadequate intake → e.g. Nausea/vomiting/anorexia
GI loss → Loss of secretions → e.g. Diarrhoea/vomiting

Hypomagnesmia

Renal loss → Nephrotoxic chemotherapy → e.g. Platinum compounds
Renal loss → Diuretics → Loop/thiazide: inhibit absorption
Renal loss → Hypercalcaemia → Competition for transport

Figure 12.3 Tumour lysis syndrome

Potassium → Hyperkalaemia → Cardiac arrythmia, weakness, paraesthesia

Phosphate → Hyperphosphataemia → Calcium phosphate in tissues (including kidney) → Renal failure

Nucleic acid purines → (Xanthine oxidase) → Uric acid → Hyperuricaemia → Uric acid crystal formation in kidney → Renal failure

Calcium → Hypocalcaemia

Low control

Hypercalcaemia

Hypercalcaemia is the most common metabolic complication of malignancy. It can occur in up to 40% of patients with cancer and is an indicator of poor prognosis. It is particularly common in multiple myeloma, cancers of the breast, lung, kidney, head and neck, and lymphoma. In 80% of cancer-associated cases it is due to parathyroid hormone-related peptide (PTHrP) production by the tumour. PThRP acts on the bone, kidney and gastrointestinal system to increase serum calcium levels. The remaining 20% are due to local resorption of bone by osteoclasts in areas of marrow space with malignant cells.

Clinical presentation is often non-specific, and may mimic deterioration due to progressive disease (Figure 12.1). Serum calcium values should be corrected:

$$\text{corrected Ca}^{++} = \text{serum Ca}^{++} + [40 - \text{serum albumin (g/L)} \times 0.02]$$

The mainstay of treatment is rehydration using large volumes of intravenous fluids, followed by a bisphosphonate such as pamidronate. Normalisation of calcium occurs in 80% of patients but may take up to 3 days. In the remaining 20%, alternative treatments include somatostatin analogues such as octreotide, calcitonin and mithramycin. Discontinue any medication that may elevate calcium, such as thiazide diuretics.

Syndrome of inappropriate antidiuresis

Hyponatraemia is common in advanced cancer; however, the finding of concentrated urine in conjunction with hypo-osmolar plasma suggests abnormal renal free water excretion and the diagnosis of the syndrome of inappropriate antidiuresis (SIAD). This is a preferred term (to SIADH) as no ADH secretion occurs in 15% of cases. Significant symptoms occur when the serum sodium is below 125 mmol/L, and can progress to stupor, coma and seizures.

Essential criteria to establish this diagnosis are:
- plasma osmolality <275 mosmol/kg H_2O;
- plasma sodium <135 mmol/L;
- urine osmolality >100 mosmol/kg H_2O;
- normal plasma/extracellular fluid volume;
- high urinary sodium (urine sodium >20 mmol/L).

Supportive criteria for this diagnosis are:
- abnormal water load test (unable to excrete >90% of a 20 mL/kg water load in 4 h, and/or failure to dilute urine to osmolality <100 mosmol/kg H_2O);
- elevated plasma arginine vasopressin levels.

In euvolaemic hyponatraemia, treatment is with fluid restriction and domeclocycline. Hypertonic saline can be used if the onset of symptoms was rapid or severe. A loop diuretic may help correct hyponatraemia but should be used with caution. Treatment of the underlying cancer may reduce ectopic ADH secretion and improve the patient's symptoms.

Hypomagnesaemia

Hypomagnesaemia usually occurs due to loss from the gastrointestinal or renal tract. There is concurrent hypokalaemia in up to 60% of cases due to shared mechanisms of loss, such as diarrhoea. In severe hypomagnesaemia (<0.5 mmol/L), there is hypocalcaemia, as PTH secretion is stimulated in the presence of low magnesium.

Patients present with a range of symptoms related to neuromuscular and neurological excitability and cardiac arrhythmia. Symptoms can be due to concurrent hypokalaemia and hypocalcaemia, and patients may have a metabolic acidosis. Patients may be irritable, disorientated and experience episodes of psychosis, seizure and even coma. Arrhythmias are common if there is pre-existing heart disease.

Serum biochemistry, including calcium, creatinine and ionised magnesium, should be measured as a proportion of magnesium is bound to plasma proteins at any one time.

The rate of correction will depend on the severity of symptoms and patients may require a slow intravenous dose of 50 mmol over 8 to 24 hours. Magnesium is slow to correct in cells and an abrupt rise in serum magnesium concentration, which is the regulator of magnesium reabsorption in the Loop of Henlé, will cause a switch to magnesium excretion and a high proportion of the treatment given will be lost. Therefore once a patient is asymptomatic, oral sustained release therapy should be given.

Tumour lysis syndrome

The acute destruction of a large number of cells is associated with metabolic sequelae, and is called tumour lysis syndrome. It is associated with bulky, chemosensitive disease including lymphoma, leukaemia and germ cell tumours when metastatic. More rarely, it can occur spontaneously. Cellular destruction results in the release of potassium, phosphate, nucleic acids and purines, which can cause transient hypocalcaemia, hyperphosphataemia, hyperuricaemia and hyperkalaemia. The release of calcium and phosphate into the bloodstream rarely causes any significant consequences. However, the calcium and phosphate may co-precipitate and cause some impairment of renal function. Nucleic acid breakdown leads to hyperuricaemia and this, unless treated appropriately, can be complicated by renal failure due to the precipitation of uric acid crystals in the renal tubular system.

Patients develop acute renal failure and present with symptoms associated with multiple underlying electrolyte abnormalities, including fatigue, nausea, vomiting, cardiac arrhythmia, heart failure, syncope, tetany, seizures and sudden death.

Serum biochemistry should be monitored regularly for 48–72 hours after treatment in patients at risk. Elevated serum potassium may be the earliest biochemical marker, but pre-treatment LDH correlates with tumour bulk and may indicate increased risk. Good hydration and urine output should be maintained throughout treatment administration. Prophylaxis with allopurinol should be considered and recombinant urate oxidase (rasburicase) can be used to reduce uric acid levels when other treatments fail. Adequate hydration is vital as it has a dilution effect on the extracellular fluid, improving electrolyte imbalance, and increases circulating volume, improving filtration in the kidneys. In high-risk patients, hydration should be commenced 24 hours before the start of treatment.

Urinary alkalisation is not routine but may be used alongside careful monitoring to reduce uric acid crystal formation. If normal treatment methods fail to correct problems, haemodialysis should be considered at an early stage to prevent progression to irreversible renal failure.

Figure 13.1 Clinical features of oncological emergencies

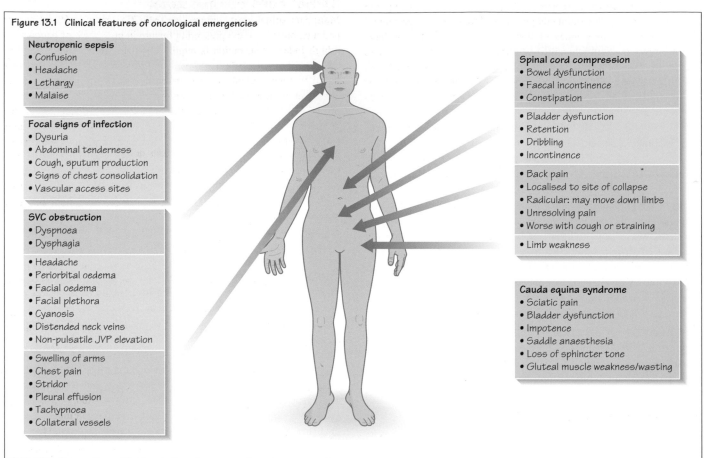

Neutropenic sepsis
- Confusion
- Headache
- Lethargy
- Malaise

Focal signs of infection
- Dysuria
- Abdominal tenderness
- Cough, sputum production
- Signs of chest consolidation
- Vascular access sites

SVC obstruction
- Dyspnoea
- Dysphagia

- Headache
- Periorbital oedema
- Facial oedema
- Facial plethora
- Cyanosis
- Distended neck veins
- Non-pulsatile JVP elevation

- Swelling of arms
- Chest pain
- Stridor
- Pleural effusion
- Tachypnoea
- Collateral vessels

Spinal cord compression
- Bowel dysfunction
- Faecal incontinence
- Constipation

- Bladder dysfunction
- Retention
- Dribbling
- Incontinence

- Back pain
- Localised to site of collapse
- Radicular: may move down limbs
- Unresolving pain
- Worse with cough or straining

- Limb weakness

Cauda equina syndrome
- Sciatic pain
- Bladder dysfunction
- Impotence
- Saddle anaesthesia
- Loss of sphincter tone
- Gluteal muscle weakness/wasting

Table 13.1 Comparison of features of cord, conus and cauda compression

Clinical feature	Spinal cord	Conus medullaris	Cauda equina
Weakness	Symmetrical and profound	Symmetrical and variable	Asymmetrical, may be mild
Reflexes	Increased or absent knee and ankle extensor plantar reflex	Increased knee, decreased ankle extensor plantar reflex	Decreased knee and ankle extensor plantar reflex
Sensory loss	Symmetrical, sensory level	Symmetrical, saddle distribution	Asymmetrical, radicular pattern
Sphincters	Late loss	Early loss	Spared often
Progression	Rapid	Variable	Variable

Figure 13.2 Approach to neutropenic sepsis

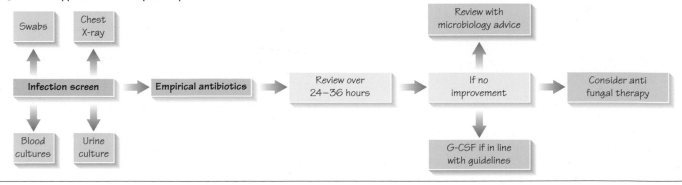

Swabs

Chest X-ray

Review with microbiology advice

Infection screen → Empirical antibiotics → Review over 24–36 hours → If no improvement → Consider anti fungal therapy

Blood cultures

Urine culture

G-CSF if in line with guidelines

Neutropenic sepsis

Neutropenia is defined as a neutrophil count of $<0.5 \times 10^9$/L, which is a common treatment-related toxicity. When associated with a fever of $>38°C$ it is known as febrile neutropenia. Infection can rapidly progress to fatality, so prompt recognition and treatment is paramount. There should be a high index of suspicion in all patients who have recently received chemotherapy, and although there are other causes of fever in the cancer patient, infection should always be assumed until proven otherwise. Neutropenia can occur following radiotherapy if large volumes of bone marrow are irradiated, or may be part of pancytopenia due to malignant infiltration of the marrow.

Initial management should include an infection screen comprising: blood cultures (peripheral and from central line if present), MSU, chest X-ray and swabs for culture (e.g. throat, central line site). No additional microbiological assessments are of benefit in the absence of localising signs of infection.

The standard approach is then to commence empirical antibiotics according to local hospital policies agreed with the microbiologists and based on the local antibiotic resistance patterns observed. First-line empirical therapy is either monotherapy with tazocin or meropenem, or with the addition of gentamicin. Metronidazole may be added if anaerobic infection is suspected, and flucloxicillin, vancomycin or teicoplanin if Gram-positive infection is suspected. Antibiotics should be adjusted according to culture results, although these are often negative. If there is no response after 36–48 hours, antibiotics should be reviewed with microbiological advice and antifungal cover should be considered. G-CSF is not routinely used for all patients with neutropenia and guidelines for use have been established.

Superior vena cava obstruction

Obstruction of the superior vena cava (SVC) by mediastinal tumours occurs most frequently with lung cancers, especially SCLC, but also with lymphoma, germ cell tumours and metastasis from other tumours. It may also be caused by a thrombus, especially in patients with a central intravenous catheter.

Presentation is commonly insidious, over weeks to months as a tumour enlarges, although it can occur more acutely. Symptoms include: headaches; dusky skin coloration over the chest, arms and face; oedema of the arms and face; and distended neck and arm veins. Other features include laryngeal or glossal oedema, mental status changes and pleural effusion (more commonly right-sided).

The severity relates to the rate of obstruction and the presence of compensatory venous collateral circulation. The flow of blood in collaterals can help confirm the clinical diagnosis. An important clinical feature is an elevated but non-pulsatile JVP. The patient may seem breathless at rest or have audible stridor. The main investigation is CT imaging of the chest with contrast.

The patient should be sat upright and breathlessness treated with oxygen. Opioids may be used for pain and may relieve dyspnoea. High-dose steroid therapy with dexamethasone should be started to reduce oedema around the tumour.

A tissue diagnosis should be made urgently if at all possible, as some tumours that can cause SVC obstruction are better treated with chemotherapy than radiotherapy (e.g. lymphoma, germ-cell tumour). For most tumours the optimal treatment is stenting of the SVC followed by mediastinal radiotherapy, which relieves symptoms in up to 90% of patients within 2 weeks.

Spinal cord compression

Malignant spinal cord compression (MSCC) occurs in 5% of cancer patients, but can be the presenting feature in up to 20% of patients, so a high index of suspicion is required both in known patients and in others with persisting symptoms. Compression may be due to a vertebral tumour, collapse of a vertebra due to tumour destruction, or a tumour of the cord itself. Intramedullary spinal cord metastases produce oedema, distortion and compression of the spinal cord parenchyma, resulting in symptoms and signs that are similar to epidural spinal cord compression. It is most common in primary cancers of bone or those that metastasise to bone, such as breast, prostate and lung cancers, and multiple myeloma.

Compression occurs commonly by posterior expansion of vertebral metastases or extension of paraspinal metastases through the intervertebral foramina. It is located in the thoracic spine in 70%, the lumbar spine in 20% and cervical spine in 10% of cases.

The earliest symptom of cord compression is vertebral pain, especially on coughing and lying flat. Signs include sensory changes one or two dermatomes below the level of compression, progressing to motor weakness distal to the block and finally sphincter disturbance. Distal compression may cause conus medullaris or caudal equina compression (Table 13.1). The finding of bilateral upper motor neurone signs should be considered spinal cord compression until proved otherwise.

Spinal cord compression should be treated as a medical emergency and the patient started on high-dose steroid therapy (dexamethasone 16 mg IV and 8 mg BD orally). An urgent MRI scan should be performed and discussed with the neurosurgeons. Plain film X-rays can show vertebral collapse but may miss up to 20% of cases.

Management is based on fast recognition and response to prevent progression to irreversible neurological problems. Surgical decompression is appropriate in patients with one site of cord compression and very limited disease in the spine or elsewhere. If this is their first presentation of cancer, histology can be obtained at surgery. Other indications for surgery are skeletal instability or recurrent compression following radiotherapy in patients without extensive metastatic disease.

In other patients, urgent radiotherapy should be given, although symptoms may worsen before they improve due to radiation-induced oedema. Response to non-surgical therapy and the duration of survival following treatment can vary considerably among different tumour types.

The degree of pre-treatment neurological dysfunction is the strongest predictor of treatment outcome. Ambulation can be preserved in more than 80% of patients who are ambulatory at presentation, but paraplegia, quadriplegia and loss of bowel or bladder function are potential consequences of cord compression if it is diagnosed late or left untreated, and once lost, neurological function cannot be regained in the majority of patients.

Approximately 30% of patients will survive for 1 year and the key to successful management is a heightened awareness of signs and symptoms, specifically new-onset back pain or motor dysfunction, leading to early diagnosis and treatment.

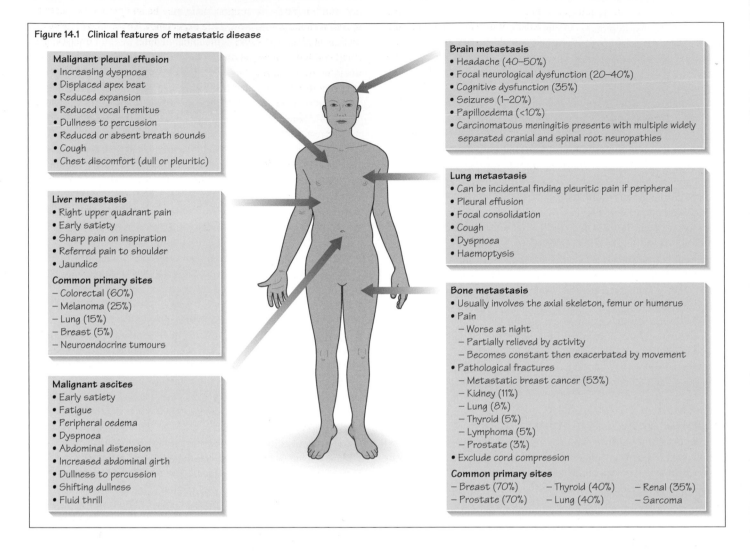

Figure 14.1 Clinical features of metastatic disease

Malignant pleural effusion
• Increasing dyspnoea
• Displaced apex beat
• Reduced expansion
• Reduced vocal fremitus
• Dullness to percussion
• Reduced or absent breath sounds
• Cough
• Chest discomfort (dull or pleuritic)

Liver metastasis
• Right upper quadrant pain
• Early satiety
• Sharp pain on inspiration
• Referred pain to shoulder
• Jaundice
Common primary sites
– Colorectal (60%)
– Melanoma (25%)
– Lung (15%)
– Breast (5%)
– Neuroendocrine tumours

Malignant ascites
• Early satiety
• Fatigue
• Peripheral oedema
• Dyspnoea
• Abdominal distension
• Increased abdominal girth
• Dullness to percussion
• Shifting dullness
• Fluid thrill

Brain metastasis
• Headache (40–50%)
• Focal neurological dysfunction (20–40%)
• Cognitive dysfunction (35%)
• Seizures (1–20%)
• Papilloedema (<10%)
• Carcinomatous meningitis presents with multiple widely separated cranial and spinal root neuropathies

Lung metastasis
• Can be incidental finding pleuritic pain if peripheral
• Pleural effusion
• Focal consolidation
• Cough
• Dyspnoea
• Haemoptysis

Bone metastasis
• Usually involves the axial skeleton, femur or humerus
• Pain
  – Worse at night
  – Partially relieved by activity
  – Becomes constant then exacerbated by movement
• Pathological fractures
  – Metastatic breast cancer (53%)
  – Kidney (11%)
  – Lung (8%)
  – Thyroid (5%)
  – Lymphoma (5%)
  – Prostate (3%)
• Exclude cord compression
Common primary sites
– Breast (70%)   – Thyroid (40%)   – Renal (35%)
– Prostate (70%)   – Lung (40%)   – Sarcoma

Metastatic spread is the hallmark of malignant disease and occurs by lymphatic spread to regional lymph nodes and by haematogenous spread to distant sites. Metastatic disease is the major cause of death in patients with cancer and the principal cause of morbidity. For the majority of patients, the aim of treatment is palliative, but treatment of a solitary metastasis can occasionally be curative.

Brain metastases

Brain metastases occur in 10–30% of adults and 6–10% of children with cancer and are an important cause of morbidity. Tumours that typically metastasise to the brain include lung, breast, melanoma and colon. Most involve the brain parenchyma but can affect the cranial nerves, the blood vessels and other intracranial structures. The median survival without treatment is 1 month. Steroids can increase survival to 2–3 months and whole brain radiotherapy to 3–6 months. Patients with brain metastases as the only manifestation of an undetected

primary tumour have a median survival of 13.4 months. Tumour type influences prognosis; breast cancer has a better prognosis and colorectal cancer tends to be worse.

The diagnosis can be confirmed by CT imaging or contrast-enhanced MRI. Carcinomatous meningitis can be confirmed by finding malignant cells in the CSF and treated with intrathecal chemotherapy. Treatment of brain metastasis includes high-dose steroids for tumour-associated oedema, anticonvulsants for seizures, whole brain radiotherapy and chemotherapy. Surgery may be considered for single sites of disease and can be curative; stereotactic radiotherapy may be considered for patients with solitary site involvement where surgery is not possible.

Lung metastases

These are common in lung, breast, colon, thyroid, sarcoma, renal, germ cell tumours and in tumours of the head and neck. Solitary lesions require investigation, as single metastases can be difficult to distinguish from primary lung tumours, although patients with two or more pulmonary nodules can be considered to have metastases.

Lung metastases are usually identified on imaging studies and the approach to treatment depends on the extent of disease in the lung and elsewhere. For solitary lesions, surgery should be considered with a generous wedge resection. Radiotherapy, chemotherapy, or endocrine therapy can be used as systemic therapy, and treatment options are dependent on the underlying primary cancer diagnosis.

Liver metastases

Metastatic cancer in the liver can represent the sole or life-limiting component of disease for many patients with a variety of tumours. Patients are often investigated due to deranged liver function tests or an abnormality detected on imaging. In selected cases, resection of the metastasis can be contemplated, particularly if solitary. In colorectal cancer, successful resection of a metastasis improves 5-year survival from 3% to 30–40%. Other techniques such as chemoembolisation or radiofrequency ablation can be used, provided the number and size of metastases remain small. If the above approaches are not feasible, symptoms may respond to systemic chemotherapy.

Bone metastases

Bone is the third most common organ involved by metastasis, behind lung and liver. Bone metastases are an increasing management problem in other tumour types, which do not classically target to bone, due to the prolonged survival of patients. Accordingly, effective management of bony metastases has become a focus in the treatment of patients with many incurable cancers.

A sensitive method to detect bone metastases is by isotope bone scan, but this may give false-negative results in multiple myeloma due to suppression of osteoblastic activity, where plain X-rays are preferred. In patients with a solitary lesion, a biopsy is essential for a tissue diagnosis because primary bone tumours may look very similar to metastases on plain film imaging.

The aim of intervention is to achieve pain relief, preservation and restoration of function, skeletal stabilization and local tumour control (e.g. relief of tumour impingement on normal structure). Surgical intervention may be warranted where there is evidence of skeletal instability (e.g. anterior or posterior spinal column fracture) or an impending fracture (e.g. large lytic lesion on a weight-bearing joint). Intravenous bisphosphonates (pamidronate, zolendronic acid or ibandronate) are widely used in the treatment of patients with bone metastases and are effective at lessening pain, and in reducing further skeletal-related events such as fractures and hypercalcaemia. In certain types of cancer, such as breast and prostate, hormonal therapy may be effective. Radiotherapy, in the form of external beam therapy or systemic radionucleotides (e.g. strontium) can be useful for some patients. In cancers likely to be sensitive to chemotherapy (e.g. breast carcinoma) systemic treatment is beneficial.

Malignant pleural effusion

This is a common complication of cancer and 40% of all pleural effusions are due to malignancy. Eighty per cent of malignant pleural effusions are due to lung and breast cancer, lymphoma and leukaemia. The presence of an effusion often indicates advanced and incurable disease.

Pleural aspirate is the key investigation that may show the presence of malignant cells. Malignant effusions are commonly blood-stained and are exudates with a raised fluid/serum LDH ratio (>0.6) and a raised fluid/serum protein ratio (>0.5). Treatment should focus on the palliation of symptoms and be tailored to the patient's physical condition and prognosis. Aspiration alone may be an appropriate treatment in frail patients with a limited life expectancy. Those who present with malignant pleural effusion as the initial manifestation of breast cancer, small cell lung cancer, germ cell tumours, or lymphoma, should have the fluid aspirated and should be given systemic chemotherapy to try and treat disease in the pleural space. Treatment options for patients with recurrent pleural effusion include pleurodesis, pleurectomy and pleuroperitoneal shunt. Ideally, pleurodesis should be attempted once recurrence of effusion occurs after an initial drainage.

Malignant ascites

The collection of intraperitoneal fluid in a patient with known malignancy is most likely due to involvement of the peritoneum with serosal implants. The presence of ascites at initial diagnosis may have prognostic significance and should be investigated to demonstrate the presence of malignant cells on cytological assessment. The presence of ascites should not influence the appropriate investigation of patients as curative intent may still be possible, depending on the primary site of the cancer.

Diagnosis is usually on clinical grounds, but ultrasound, MRI, or CT imaging are useful for guided drainage, particularly where the fluid is pocketed. Non-malignant causes of ascites include congestive heart failure, liver cirrhosis, renal failure, hypoproteinemia, infectious processes and endometriosis. Approximately 10% of patients with ascites have an underlying malignancy, although in a patient with advanced cancer it is the most likely diagnosis. Investigation for cytology is indicated when a definitive diagnosis of malignant ascites is necessary for staging purposes or when planning surgical intervention. Patients with malignant ascites secondary to ovarian cancer have a significantly better outcome and therefore thorough investigation of female patients presenting with ascites of unknown origin should be undertaken.

The most common treatment is paracentesis, including the use of indwelling (Pleurx) catheters. Loop diuretics, salt restriction and aldosterone-inhibiting diuretics are generally not beneficial because sodium retention is not a cause of malignant ascites. The use of albumin has never proven beneficial in delaying fluid reaccumulation nor been more effective than crystalloid solutions in restoring intravascular volume depletion after drainage of large quantities of peritoneal fluid.

The therapeutic approaches used to treat patients with malignant ascites may include diuretics, peritoneovenous shunting, extensive surgical debulking in preparation for local or systemic or intraperitoneal chemotherapy. Although prolongation of survival has been attributed to some of these therapies, no definitive study has ever demonstrated effectiveness or superiority of any one strategy.

Other sites

Metastasis can occur at any site of the body, but the above locations are the most common in clinical practice. Skin metastasis can be uncomfortable and unsightly for some patients, and local radiotherapy can provide control in some cases.

Involvement of the heart is very unusual, but pericardial disease and effusions are seen in breast, lung and ovarian cancer, which account for 75% of cases. Management is similar to that for malignant ascites, with drainage and systemic treatment for the underlying cancer.

Table 15.1 Examples of serum tumour markers

Tumour marker	Related cancers
β2-microglobulin	Myeloma (60%) Non-Hodgkin's lymphoma (15%)
Alpha-fetoprotein (AFP)	Non-seminomatous germ cell tumours (80%) Hepatocellular carcinoma (50%)
CA125	Ovarian epithelial cancer (80%) Gastrointestinal cancer (10%) Breast cancer (5%) Lung cancer (5%)
CA15-3	Breast cancer
CA19-9	Pancreatic cancer (80%) Mucinous tumour of the ovary (65%) Gastric cancer (30%) Colon cancer (30%)
Calcitonin	Medullary cell carcinoma of the thyroid
Carcinoembryonic antigen (CEA)	Colorectal cancer (especially with liver metastasis) Gastric cancer Breast cancer Lung cancer
Human chorionic gonadotrophin (β-hCG)	Choriocarcinoma (100%) Non-seminomatous germ cell tumours (50–80%) Seminoma (15%)
Inhibin	Granulosa cell cancer of the ovary
Neurone-specific enolase	Neuroblastoma Small cell lung cancer
Paraproteins (monoclonal)	Myeloma (98%)
Placental alkaline phosphatase (PLAP)	Seminoma (50%) Ovarian dysgerminoma (50%)
Prostate-specific antigen (PSA)	Prostate cancer (95%)
SCC	Squamous cell cervical cancer Squamous head and neck cancer
Thyroglobulin	Papillary and follicular thyroid cancer

Serum proteins

Tumour markers are secreted proteins produced by cancers that are detectable in the serum of patients. Some have found clinical application as a means of monitoring the course of disease and as prognostic factors. Tumour markers may be used for population screening, diagnosis, prognostic factors, monitoring treatment, diagnosis of relapse and imaging of metastases. The minimal requirements for a tumour marker are:

- reliable, quick, cheap assay;
- high sensitivity (>50%) and specificity (>95%);
- high predictive value of positive and negative results.

Clinical usefulness

The *sensitivity* of a test is defined as the percentage of patients with a particular disease who have elevated marker levels and are therefore true positives. *Specificity* is the percentage of patients without disease who have normal marker levels and are therefore true negatives. The *positive predictive value* is the percentage of positive results (i.e. elevated marker levels) that are true positives. The false-positive rate is the percentage of patients without disease who have an elevated marker level. The false-negative rate is the percentage of patients with disease who have a normal marker level.

Human chorionic gonadotrophin

Human chorionic gonadotrophin (hCG) is a glycoprotein formed physiologically in the syncytiotrophoblast of the placenta, which is used to diagnose and monitor pregnancy, gestational trophoblastic disease and germ cell tumours. The sensitivity is 100% for testicular and placental choriocarcinomas and hydatidiform moles, 48–86% for NSGCT and 7–14% for seminomas. This is the closest model to a perfect tumour marker.

Alpha-fetoprotein

Alpha-fetoprotein (AFP) is synthesised by fetal yolk sac, liver and intestine, and in the fetus is the major serum protein acting as an albumin-like carrier protein. Moderately elevated levels are seen in some patients with pancreatic, biliary, gastric and bronchial cancers, as well as occasional patients with non-malignant hepatic disease where active hepatic regeneration is occurring. Increased levels are found in patients with hepatocellular carcinoma and GCT of the testes, ovary and midline structures, including mediastinum and pineal gland, that contain yolk sac tissue. Serum values occasionally increase as a result of chemotherapy.

Placental alkaline phosphatase

An isoenzyme of alkaline phosphatase is elevated in testicular seminoma and ovarian dysgerminoma, but slightly elevated serum levels are found in people who smoke.

CA19-9

CA19-9 is a mucin found in epithelium of fetal stomach, intestine and pancreas. Its main use is to monitor response to treatment in gastric and pancreatic cancer. Levels do not generally correspond well to tumour bulk, although levels above 10000 mostly indicate the presence of metastatic disease. It is not useful in screening for pancreatic cancer. CA19-9 is eliminated exclusively via bile. Any degree of cholestasis can cause levels to rise. It can be elevated in mucinous tumours of the ovary.

Inhibin

Inhibin is a protein secreted by granulosa cells including Sertoli cells and it inhibits pituitary FSH secretion. It is a more useful marker than oestradiol in monitoring the rare granulosa cell tumours of the ovary.

Carcinoembryonic antigen (CEA)

This glycoprotein is elevated in carcinomas of the gastrointestinal tract and fetal digestive organs, and also in a variety of other malignant and non-malignant conditions. These include severe benign liver disease, inflammatory lesions (particularly of the gastrointestinal tract), infections, trauma, infarction, collagen diseases, renal impairment and smoking. Low values are also found in the normal colon. Patients with widespread metastases from tumours, including breast, stomach, bronchus, pancreas, oesophagus, cervix, ovary and endometrium, may have elevated serum CEA levels, which can be used to monitor the response to treatment.

CA15-3

Elevated serum levels of CA15-3 have been found in 12.5% of women with benign breast disease, in 11% of women with operable breast cancer and in 64% of women with metastatic breast cancer. The mucin-like carcinoma-associated antigen has no role in screening because of the low sensitivity for early stages of the disease. It can be elevated in some patients with gynaecological cancers. CA15-3 elevation increases with increasing stage of disease and the highest levels are seen in patients with liver or bone metastases. A rising CA15-3 level during follow-up can detect relapse 2–9 months before clinical signs or symptoms develop.

CA125

CA125 is produced from derivatives of the coelomic epithelium, including the pleura, pericardium, peritoneum, fallopian tube, endometrium and endocervix. It has been detected in many tissues and secretions, but not in the normal ovary. The antigen is present at the cell surface in more than 80% of non-mucinous epithelial ovarian tumours and in a small percentage of other tumours. However, this is elevated in more than 90% of patients with stage III or IV disease but in only 50% with stage I disease. More than 40% of patients with advanced intra-abdominal cancers of diverse primary site and histology have elevated levels of CA125.

CA125 has a low sensitivity for stage I tumours, suggesting that it is unlikely to have a role in screening, but this is being investigated with a clinical trial. Very high CA125 levels prior to surgery are associated with a worse prognosis. However, the most important prognostic factors are: the CA125 level after one, two, or three courses of chemotherapy; a short half-life; or greater than sevenfold fall in CA125. It is therefore useful in the monitoring of response to chemotherapy for ovarian cancer and for detection of relapse.

Squamous cell carcinoma-associated antigen (SCC)

SCC is a glycoprotein that is mainly used for monitoring treatment of squamous cell cervical cancer (sensitivity 70–85%) and of head and neck squamous carcinomas (sensitivity 60%). Elevated levels are found in 17% of all NSCLC and in 31% of squamous NSCLC.

Prostate-specific antigen (PSA)

PSA is a serine protease produced by prostate epithelium with the function of liquefying the gel that surrounds spermatozoa to enable them to become fully mobile. Elevated serum levels of PSA (>4 ng/mL) occur in 50% of men with intracapsular microscopic prostate cancer and 77% of men with intracapsular macroscopic disease. It is seen in 30–50% of men with benign prostatic hypertrophy.

The combination of PSA and digital rectal examination, followed by prostatic ultrasound in patients with abnormal findings, is commonly used for screening in the USA but is not recommended in the UK as there is no evidence of survival benefit from early detection of prostate cancer.

Hormones

Several tumours of endocrine tissue can be diagnosed and treatment monitored by serial measurement. Calcitonin and calcitonin gene-related peptide are used in screening for medullary carcinoma of the thyroid. Catecholamine metabolites, vanillylmandelic acid and homovanillic acid can be used to detect neuroblastoma.

Table 16.1 World Health Organization considerations for successful screening

1.	The population to screen should be agreed
2.	The test should be acceptable
3.	Screening is for a condition of importance
4.	Latent period allows for intervention
5.	The disease natural history is well understood
6.	Diagnostic facilities are available
7.	Appropriate test is available
8.	Effective early treatment is available
9.	The programme is cost effective
10.	Screening should be continuous, i.e. screening and treatment of the condition does not result in eradication and therefore testing is required from one generation to the next

Table 16.2 Utility of a screening test

Specificity: ability to detect negatives	=	true negatives/ true negatives + false positives
Specificity: ability to detect positives	=	true positives/ true positives + false negatives
Positive predictive value	=	true positives/ true positives + false positives
Negative predictive value	=	true negatives/ true negatives + false negatives

Table 16.3 Factors to consider when assessing a screening programme

- Is the disease curable if diagnosed early?
- What is the sensitivity of the test used?
- Is the disease common?
- How frequently should the test be done?
- What population should be tested?
- What are the disadvantages of screening?

Cancer screening describes the systematic testing of a population in order to detect a cancer before it causes symptoms. The World Health Organization has identified key features that are required for successful screening (Table 16.1). These relate to the tribe (population), test, treatment, tumour and treasury (money). Unfortunately, there are few cancers for which population screening is available.

The utility of a screening test depends on the ability to detect a true positive (sensitivity) and the ability to reject a true negative (specificity) (Table 16.2).

Successful screening

For screening to be successful the detection test should be easy to use and should ideally detect a pre-cancerous condition that allows treat-ment before the development of an invasive cancer. There are few cancers that have a natural history that allows detection of a pre-cancerous condition. There should be a clearly defined target population and increasingly this will be defined on the basis of molecular abnormalities such as *BRCA1* gene status for breast and ovarian cancer, or *APC* gene status for colorectal cancer. In such target groups the higher risk is matched by more intensive screening, or alternatively the opportunity to intervene to reduce risk using prophylactic surgery with mastectomy, oophorectomy or colectomy.

Successful detection has to be coupled to an intervention that changes the natural history of the cancer and offers extension of lifespan. The more advanced the cancer at the point of detection, the smaller the magnitude of intervention that will impact on survival. For some patients there is a resistance to attend for screening, and education of the population about the benefits is key.

Lead time bias
The introduction of screening can detect tumours at an earlier (pre-symptomatic) stage, therefore when compared with a symptomatic cohort the subsequent survival is spuriously prolonged, even if earlier treatment does not actually increase lifespan. For screening to be beneficial, the earlier detection and treatment must impact on mortality, increasing lifespan.

Length time bias
Slower-growing cancers have a longer latent period and are more likely to be detected by screening. At the start of a screening programme more patients with indolent disease will be detected, because at any one time the prevalence of slowly growing tumours will be greater even if the incidence of aggressive tumours is similar. This bias leads to an illusory survival improvement in the screened cohort. The improved survival time of these patients cannot wholly be attributed to earlier treatment.

Breast cancer screening
Mammographic screening represents an important advance in the management of breast cancer. A large percentage of screening-detected cancers are less than 2 cm without axillary nodal spread, or are in situ tumours only. The suspicious mammographic features are microcalcification and soft tissue density within the breast.

Some randomised population-based trials showed a reduction of 25% in breast cancer mortality. The age groups found to benefit were age 50–69 years; older women have not been adequately assessed. A benefit in younger women has not been proven. Most interval cancers occur in the third year after screening suggesting that the optimal frequency may be every 2 years. In the UK, women aged 50–70 years are offered two-view mammographic screening every 3 years.

Colorectal cancer screening
Four randomised controlled studies have shown that population screening of people over 50 years old for faecal occult blood reduces colorectal cancer deaths. Case-control studies have shown that sigmoidoscopy is effective for population screening. A pilot screening programme is underway in the UK. Members of families with FAP or HNPCC should have surveillance colonoscopy every 1–3 years, which reduces deaths from colon cancer.

Gastric cancer screening
Gastric cancer is surgically curable if detected early and in Japan, where the incidence is high, endoscopic screening has increased the number of cancers that are detected at an early stage and are cured.

Prostate cancer screening
An early screening trial of serum PSA measurement and digital rectal examination in 18 000 men detected a cancer rate of 3.5%, of which more than 90% were localised tumours that were amenable to radical curative therapy. This led to interest in a prostate cancer screening programme, particularly in the USA. However, no randomised controlled trials have adequately addressed the impact of screening on survival. This is perhaps not surprising because no randomised clinical trials have evaluated the optimal therapy for localised early prostate cancer either. Models of screening reveal part of the reason for this: 3% of men are expected to die of prostate cancer and the average life reduction is 9 years. Thus, for 100 men an ideal screening programme coupled to a complete curative therapy could prevent three deaths and gain 27 years of life. This translates to an increased life expectancy for the whole screened cohort of 3 months.

Cervical cancer screening
Exfoliative cytology and Papanicolaou staining form the basis of cervical smear screening for the detection of premalignant cervical intraepithelial neoplasia (CIN). The cervical screening programme has reduced the incidence of squamous cancer of the cervix but is not able to reliably detect adenocarcinoma.

Abnormal smears (CIN 2/3) should be followed by colposcopy (visualisation of the cervix under 10–15 power magnification with bright light and green filter to enhance vascular pattern) and biopsy. If colposcopic biopsy is incomplete, patients should proceed to cone biopsy, removing the transition zone. In the UK, women aged 25–49 years are offered screening every 3 years and women aged 50–64 years are screened 5-yearly.

Ovarian cancer screening
Ovarian screening by serum CA125 tumour marker measurement and/or transvaginal ultrasound is under investigation in randomised clinical trials. Although this approach is feasible and can detect tumours at an earlier and more treatable stage, there is as yet no evidence of improved survival in screened cohorts. Even in women with *BRCA1* or *BRCA2* mutations there is no evidence to support screening.

Lung cancer screening
Screening for lung cancer by chest radiograph and/or sputum cytology has not been found to be effective, even in high-risk populations. Four randomised trials have failed to show a reduction in lung cancer mortality. Low-dose helical CT scans for detecting early lung cancers are still under evaluation.

The future
Successful screening requires better detection methods coupled to better treatments. Furthermore, developments in molecular medicine have greatly increased the understanding of the development of cancer and have led to the characterisation of a large number of cancer predisposition syndromes. Patients with an indentified risk due to a genetic abnormality may have the opportunity for preventative intervention, but such patients are often underserved by existing provision and the cancers can develop at an age before National Screening Programmes begin.

Only approximately 10% of all adult cancers are due to a genetic predisposition and further study is needed to establish efficacious screening protocols for those who are not genetically predisposed to cancer.

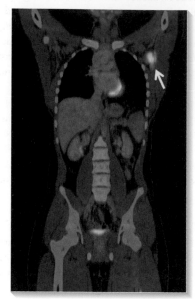

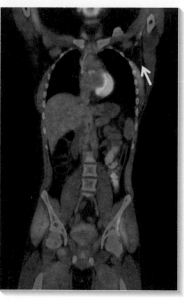

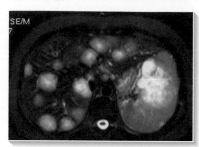

Figure 17.3
MRI scan showing liver metastasis from ovarian cancer

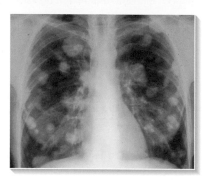

Figure 17.4
A chest X-ray showing multiple lung metastases

Figure 17.1
A PET scan showing a positive lymph node in the left axilla. Normal uptake is seen in the heart and bladder

Figure 17.2
A repeat PET image following treatment showing resolution of the lymph node

Table 17.1 Interventional radiology approaches in oncology practice

Central indwelling catheter	Indwelling catheters are inserted under ultrasound guidance into the subclavian vein and into the right atrium. They can be used for vascular access, sampling blood and delivery of chemotherapy
Chemoembolisation	Occlusion of an artery to induce ischaemia and resulting tumour necrosis, and to arrest growth by the intra-arterial delivery of particulate materials, sclerosing solutions or liquid that solidifies. This can be used to control bleeding, particularly GI haemorrhage, to facilitate surgical resection by decreasing blood loss and operating time, to inhibit tumour growth and to relieve pain by decreasing tumour bulk
Focused ultrasound	A converging, high-intensity, focused ultrasound beam can be applied to treat tumour tissue, particularly if deeply embedded. The localised high temperature induces cell damage due to protein denaturation and capillary bed destruction, causing subsequent coagulation necrosis that occurs without injuring the surrounding non-targeted tissue. It is particularly useful in the treatment of liver metastasis
Image-guided biopsy	Percutaneous biopsy is a cost-effective approach to diagnosis of cancer. Almost all tissues are accessible to percutaneous biopsy, which can be achieved as an outpatient using sedation and local analgesia
Mechanical devices	Ureteric stents, colonic and biliary stents are all examples of where a radiologist can significantly improve symptoms in a patient with obstruction of a conduit
Oesophageal stent	Stent insertion for oesophageal obstruction can restore function and quality of life in patients with malignant obstruction due to a circumferential lesion or extrinsic compression
Vena cava filter	Patients with cancer have a particularly high risk of thromboembolism and patients can have a filter inserted into the IVC to reduce the risk of pulmonary emboli. This is particularly useful for patients considered for surgery who cannot remain on full anticoagulation
Venous stent	Used to recannulate the SVC following obstruction from an extrinsic mass

Imaging is a key service required for the delivery of cancer care, from obtaining a diagnosis, to determining the extent of disease, assessing response to treatments, detecting recurrent disease and the use of interventional approaches (Table 17.1). It is important to consider whether a particular test will influence the management of a patient and this should be balanced against the potential harm of exposure to ionising radiation used in some forms of imaging.

Plain film imaging

Plain films are particularly useful for imaging the skeleton. They can demonstrate sclerotic and lytic bone reactions due to metastasis and provide information about the likelihood for an impending fracture due to metastatic disease. A chest X-ray is a simple means of screening for metastasis to the lungs and for suspected infection.

Plain film imaging is used for mammographic screening of women for breast cancer. This is a radiological investigation for lumps and microcalcifications. Both invasive cancers and ductal carcinoma in situ can be detected using this imaging modality. Women testing positive are referred for assessment with clinical examination, ultrasound and FNA cytology. Mammography remains the only imaging method clearly proven effective when applied in the screening setting.

Ultrasound

Ultrasound imaging can be performed at the bedside. Through the use of high-frequency sound waves images can be obtained in many planes, but this is reliant on a skilled operator. The sound waves do not penetrate well into areas of gas or bone and are reflected, causing a 'shadow effect' behind the target area. The resolution is decreased by overlying fat.

Ultrasound has a clear role in screening for liver metastasis, in conjunction with clinical examination and serum biochemistry. Testicular masses can be demonstrated on ultrasound, which is effective in distinguishing cystic from solid carcinoma. This is useful when assessing thyroid, breast and particularly renal masses, where cysts can be distinguished from carcinoma in 90% of cases.

Ultrasound has been combined with endoscopy and has a role in measuring the extent of tumours of the oesophagus and bronchus.

Computerised tomography

CT is the most common imaging investigation for patients with cancer and is used to determine the extent of local invasion (T staging) as well involvement of lymph nodes or distant metastasis (N and M staging). Most cancers can benefit from CT guidance for biopsy or FNA in the diagnosis of a suspicious mass.

There are limitations, with false-positive and false-negative findings, in particular the reliability of detecting pathological lymph nodes that are approximately 1 cm in diameter or non-pathological bowel loops creating a suspicious appearance. CT is the most sensitive modality for detecting pulmonary metastasis.

Magnetic resonance imaging

MR techniques provide in vivo and in vitro anatomical, functional, physiological and molecular information about various tissues and tumours. This provides unique tissue classification through soft-tissue contrast, accurate anatomical localisation, and identification of a number of tumour and microenvironmental characteristics.

MRI is the imaging modality of choice for CNS, spinal and musculoskeletal tumours, as well as in assessing vascular, pelvic and hepatobiliary lesions where magnetic resonance cholangiopancreatography (MRCP) is becoming a popular alternative to ERCP when imaging the hepatobiliary tree. It can be used to detect breast cancers, especially in women with dense breast tissue. Recent concerns regarding gadolinium-associated nephrogenic systemic fibrosis have led to caution in the use of MRI contrast medium in patients with impaired renal function.

With faster MRI pulse sequences and greater computer storage, it is possible to track the uptake of gadolinium-DTPA and to measure tissue perfusion quantitatively with sub-millimetre resolution. In addition to perfusion, dynamic contrast-enhanced imaging can be used to measure parameters such as cerebral blood volume, blood–brain barrier permeability, necrotic fraction, extracellular space and permeability surface area product.

Radioisotope imaging

This modality has poor sensitivity and poor specificity for many tissues, but only delivers a small quantity of radiation. A bone scan uses ^{99}Technetium-labelled phosphate compounds that are taken up in areas of increased metabolic activity within the skeleton. This leads to poor specificity as the isotope is taken up in areas of infection, fracture, or metastatic disease. Therefore false-positive areas will be detected due to vertebral collapse secondary to osteoporosis, and correlation with plain film imaging is often required. Nevertheless, bone scans are a sensitive test to detect occult bone metastasis.

Radioisotopes are used in the detection of sentinel nodes during an operative procedure. The primary tumour is injected with a radiolabelled isotope and the primary lymph node draining the area is identified and removed for assessment using a Geiger counter during the procedure. This negates the requirement for a lymph node clearance when the sentinel node is negative for metastatic disease, giving a predictive power of 95%.

Positron emission tomography

PET imaging is used for preoperative staging and the monitoring of tumour response to therapy. The basis of cancer detection by FDG is the elevation of glucose metabolism by cancer cells and can differentiate between benign and malignant lesions. It has a higher sensitivity and specificity than CT for a number of cancers, e.g. NSCLC, where unsuspected metastasis is found in up to 20%, which influences choice of treatment strategy, radiotherapy planning, and is a predictor of survival.

The potential of PET to determine quantitatively the levels of accumulation of chemotherapeutic agents in tumours offers the prospect of patient-specific dosing. Furthermore, early PET responses can predict outcome from prolonged chemotherapy treatments (Figures 17.1 and 17.2). PET can be used to measure blood flow, tumour perfusion and tissue hypoxia, providing insight into the tumour microenvironment.

The fusion of anatomical and functional images to create hybrid images using PET-CT or SPECT-CT is seeing application as composite imaging for cancer diagnosis and management.

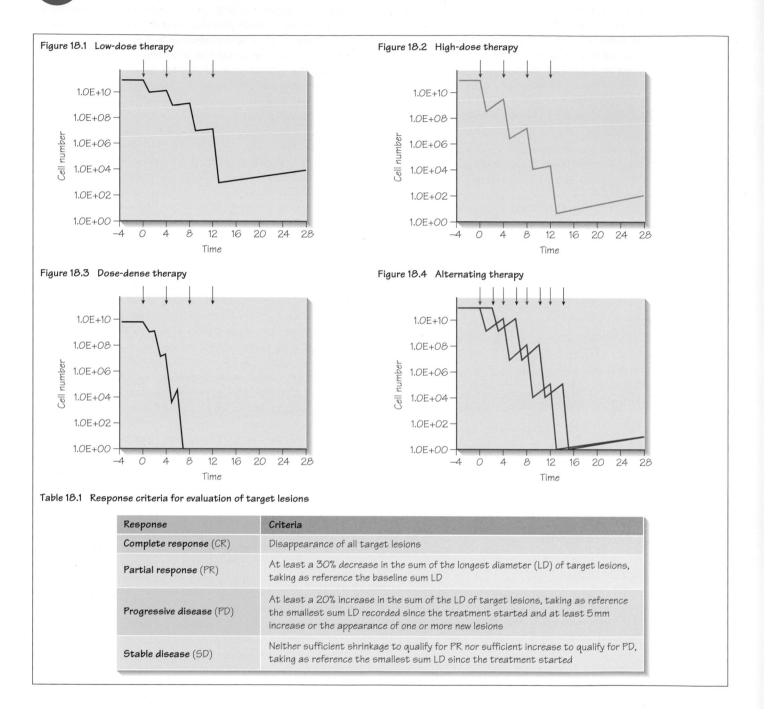

Figure 18.1 Low-dose therapy

Figure 18.2 High-dose therapy

Figure 18.3 Dose-dense therapy

Figure 18.4 Alternating therapy

Table 18.1 Response criteria for evaluation of target lesions

Response	Criteria
Complete response (CR)	Disappearance of all target lesions
Partial response (PR)	At least a 30% decrease in the sum of the longest diameter (LD) of target lesions, taking as reference the baseline sum LD
Progressive disease (PD)	At least a 20% increase in the sum of the LD of target lesions, taking as reference the smallest sum LD recorded since the treatment started and at least 5mm increase or the appearance of one or more new lesions
Stable disease (SD)	Neither sufficient shrinkage to qualify for PR nor sufficient increase to qualify for PD, taking as reference the smallest sum LD since the treatment started

Treatment goals

It is important that the goal of treatment is clear in order to manage the expectations of the patient, their relatives and the treating team. It is a requirement in the UK that the goal of treatment is recorded in the patient's medical notes. The goal can be either with curative intent or for palliation, and there are four main indications for therapy.

Palliative chemotherapy is indicated for the majority of patients with widespread metastasis. The goal of treatment is an improvement in symptoms with a focus on improving quality of life; survival increments are secondary. As a result the treatment should be well tolerated and aim to minimise adverse effects.

Adjuvant chemotherapy is given after an initial intervention that is designed to cytoreduce the tumour bulk and remove all macroscopic disease. Chemotherapy is then given with the intention of eradicating the micrometastatic disease that remains. The focus is on achieving an improvement in disease-free and overall survival.

Neoadjuvant chemotherapy or primary medical therapy is where chemotherapy is administered before a planned cytoreductive procedure. This can result in a reduced requirement for surgery, increase the likelihood of successful debulking, reduce the duration of hospitalisation and improve the fitness of the patient prior to interval debulking. This approach has the same goals as adjuvant treatment but creates opportunity for translational research to measure responses to treatment and correlate with subsequent specimens removed at the time of surgery.

Chemoprevention is the use of pharmacological agents to prevent cancer developing in patients identified as being at particular risk. Therefore the agents used are designed to modify risk and as such should not have significant adverse effects.

Treatment approach

The dosing schedule and interval is determined by the choice of drugs and recovery of the cancer and normal tissues. For most common chemotherapy regimens, the treatment is administered every 21 or 28 days, which defines one cycle. A course of treatment often uses up to six cycles of treatment. An increase in effectiveness can be achieved by changing the approach to treatment. In some cases this will increase toxicity too, but it can change the nature of the toxicity and such developments are evaluated in clinical trials.

Low-dose therapy is the standard approach and most palliative chemotherapy is given in this manner. The next cycle is started once the bone marrow function has recovered sufficiently to start the treatment (neutrophils $>1.0 \times 10^9$/L and platelets $>100 \times 10^9$/L).

High-dose therapy uses a higher individual drug dose to achieve a higher cell kill but results in more bone marrow toxicity. This can be minimised by using G-CSF. This approach allows more drug to be delivered within the same schedule of administration but the total received dose can be less than the intended dose due to limitations of non-haematological toxicity.

Dose-dense therapy involves fractionating the intended dose of drug and administering each fraction on a more frequent basis (often weekly). Each individual dose produces less toxicity but the anticancer effect is related to the cumulative dose over time. Such an approach can overcome drug resistance, produce a greater cell kill and in some cases produce a response with weekly administration when the 3-weekly schedule demonstrates a lack of response or even disease progression.

Alternating therapy involves giving different drugs in an alternating manner. This is most commonly used with haematological malignancies and is designed to treat different subpopulations of cancer cells where individual clones of cells might be resistant to one or more of the agents.

Assessment of toxicity

Most anticancer treatment is given at the maximum dose tolerated by the patient and adverse effects are inevitable. There are common toxicity criteria (CTC) scales that rate the severity of several hundred side effects on a four-point scale. This allows an objective measurement and comparison over time throughout treatment. Detailed information ad the current version of the CTC is maintained by the National Cancer Institute and is available at http://ctep.cancer.gov/reporting/ctc.html.

Evaluation of treatment

The evaluation of treatments includes an assessment of overall survival duration, response to treatment, remission rate, disease-free survival and response duration, quality of life and treatment toxicity.

Uniform criteria have been established to measure these, including the response evaluation criteria in solid tumours (RECIST) (Table 15.1). This allows clinicians to accurately inform patients of the prognosis, effectiveness and toxicity of chemotherapy, and empowers patients to take an active role in treatment decisions.

Overall survival rate is the percentage of patients in a study or treatment group who are alive for a certain period of time after the diagnosis of cancer. This is usually stated as a 5-year survival rate, which is the percentage of patients in a defined group who are alive 5 years after diagnosis or treatment.

Remission rate is the percentage of patients who achieve a state where the cancer is no longer detectable. This is complete remission where all signs and symptoms of cancer have disappeared, although cancer may still be in the body. In partial remission, some, but not all, signs and symptoms of cancer have disappeared.

Disease-free survival is the length of time after treatment for cancer during which a patient survives with no symptoms or signs of the disease. Disease-free survival may be used in a clinical trial to measure how well a new treatment works.

Response is usually assessed in accordance with the RECIST 1.1 criteria with pre-treatment documentation of target and non-target lesions. All measurable lesions up to a maximum of two lesions per organ and five lesions in total, representative of all involved organs, should be identified as target lesions and measured at baseline. Target lesions should be selected on the basis of their size (lesions with the longest diameter) and their suitability for accurate repeated measurements (either by imaging techniques or clinically). A sum of the longest diameter (LD) for all target lesions will be calculated and recorded as the baseline sum LD, used as a reference to characterise the objective response. All other lesions (or sites of disease) should be identified as non-target lesions and be recorded at baseline.

Measurable disease is defined as at least one lesion that can be accurately measured in at least one dimension (longest diameter [LD] to be recorded). Each lesion must be >10 mm when assessed by CT and MRI (if the slice thickness is ≤5 mm), and clinical examination; or >20 mm when measured by plain X-ray. (For CT and MRI scans where the slice thickness is >5 mm, measurability is defined as a lesion with LD > 2x the slice thickness.) For malignant lymph nodes, short axis diameter must by >15 mm to be considered pathological and measurable.

Non-measurable disease includes aspects that are more subjective in their assessment and based on factors such as tumour marker levels, presence of ascites, or effusions.

Residual disease is that left at completion of planned treatment and, if present, indicates resistance to the treatment and is therefore an adverse prognostic factor. In some circumstances it may be difficult to distinguish residual disease from normal tissue, particularly in patients with postoperative changes following abdominal or pelvic surgery. When the evaluation of complete response depends on this determination, it is recommended that the residual lesion be investigated (fine needle aspirate/biopsy) to confirm the complete response status.

Table 19.1 Basic rules of surgical oncology

- The site and direction of skin incision for surgery with curative intent should be appropriate to allow adequate removal of the primary tumour and debulking of disease
- The tumour and associated lymph nodes should be removed with clear margins of normal tissue
- Scars of biopsies should be considered contaminated with tumour and be removed en-bloc with the primary tumour
- During the surgery, instruments that might be considered contaminated with tumour cells should be replaced
- Unnecessary manipulation of the tumour should be avoided

Table 19.2 Common procedures in surgical oncology

- Excision with clear normal tissue margins
- Excision en-bloc of the primary tumour and regional lymph nodes
- Lymph node dissection
- Enucleation (less common)
- Tissue destructive methods (e.g. radiofrequency frequency ablation)
- Isolated regional perfusion
- Excision of metastasis (usually from brain, lung, liver, bone)

Table 19.3 Important characteristics in describing a lump

4 Ss	Site, Size, Surface (and overlying skin) and Secretion (any discharge from lump)
3 Cs	Colour, Contour, Consistency
3 Ts	Tenderness, Temperature, Transilluminability
3 Fs	Fluctuance, Fixation, Fields (think of draining lymph nodes in the area and surrounding tissue)
PE	If it is Pulsatile and Expansile, think aneurysm
R	If it is Reducible, think hernia
	• Remember not all lumps will have all these characteristics • Measure all lumps in centimetres in at least two dimensions

Figure 19.1 Core biopsy. Source: Dixon (2012) *ABC of Breast Diseases*, 4th edn. Wiley-Blackwell, Oxford

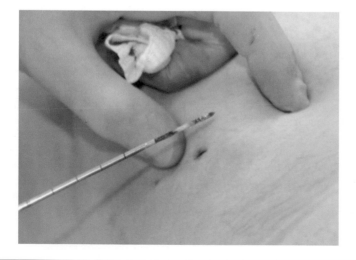

Surgical oncology

The surgical management of cancer can be dated back to the Ancient Egyptians in 1600BC, with the papyri offering the first descriptions of a cancer managed surgically. Surgeons are often involved in the initial assessment of patients and require clinical and technical skills to participate as an effective member of a multidisciplinary team (Tables 19.1 and 19.2).

Prevention

The identification of genetic predisposition syndromes allows for the intervention with prophylactic surgical removal to reduce the lifetime risk of cancer. For example: total colectomy in patients with familial adenomatous polyposis; bilateral mastectomy with reconstruction and oophorectomy for *BRCA1* and *BRCA2* gene mutation carriers; thyroidectomy for patients with multiple endocrine neoplasia to prevent medullary carcinoma of the thyroid.

Evaluation of primary disease

Adequate biopsy of any lump or mass with histological evaluation is required before starting anticancer treatment (Table 19.3). The surgeon must select an appropriate site and biopsy method, and furthermore has the responsibility to communicate the results, prognosis and treatment options effectively to the patient and their family.

Biopsy types

Fine-needle aspiration (FNA) can be performed with a 21G needle and a 20-ml syringe and can easily be repeated if there is inadequate sampling for assessment. This can be performed under image guidance, e.g. for a biopsy of liver, suspicious lymph node or breast lump. The sensitivity and specificity are >90% and false-positive rates are 0-3%. It is unsuitable for accurate diagnosis in lymphoma and inconsistent for cancers of the pancreas, thyroid and soft tissue.

Needle core biopsy (Figure 19.1) involves a cutting needle, and tissue cores obtained should be representative of the whole tumour. Deep tumours in the abdomen or retroperitoneal space can be accessed under image guidance, avoiding an open biopsy. Tumour seeding along the needle tract should be considered and is a particular problem for sarcoma.

Incision versus excision biopsy. When an open surgical biopsy is required, excision of the whole lesion is preferable to incision and sampling of only a part of the tumour. In melanoma, excision allows accurate microstaging and determination of Breslow thickness; in lymphoma, it allows identification of the architecture of the lymph node removed. In some cancers, an incision biopsy may be required when the tumour is fixed due to local extension, or previous radiotherapy producing fibrosis makes excision too hazardous. In large soft tissue tumours, an incision biopsy may cause less disruption of the tissue planes which might otherwise compromise the chances of subsequent radical surgery.

Punch biopsy removes a small fragment of superficial tumour, and while useful for superficial lesions it does not provide sufficient material for assessment of architecture and thickness.

Staging

Staging is a clinical assessment of the extent of cancer spread. It is usually a combination of surgical, histological, radiological and clinical assessments. Surgical staging techniques such as staging laparatomy or mediastinoscopy have been mostly replaced by PET/CT imaging, which avoids the morbidity of such invasive procedures.

Treatment

The aim of surgery with curative intent is to remove all macroscopic tumour with clear normal tissue margins. This can be curative for cancers confined to an organ, such as Duke's A cancers of the bowel or rectum, gastrectomy for early gastric cancer, excision of a basal cell carcinoma, or radical nephrectomy for renal cell carcinoma.

Lymph nodes are frequently removed to determine spread for staging. Lymphadenectomy can reduce the risk of metastasis and improve outcome and survival in some cancers, but at the risk of lymphoedema, which can have a significant impact on the patient. A less radical approach is a sentinel lymph node biopsy, which assumes that there is always one lymph node to which a cancer will first metastasise, and if removed and found to be clear, negates the removal of the other nodes. This can be performed using a dye or radioisotope injected at the primary cancer site and if detected in the sentinel lymph node this can be removed.

Patients who develop local recurrence can benefit from further surgical resection as maintaining local control can impact on outcome. This improves symptom control, but careful patient selection is vital. There has been a progressive abandonment of extensive mutilating surgery in favour of non-surgical options and all patients should be discussed at an appropriate multidisciplinary team meeting (MDT) (see Chapter 26).

Surgical resection of metastatic disease is considered where there is limited other disease and the number of metastases is low. Isolated metastasis to the lung, liver, or brain should be considered for removal as improvements in survival have been demonstrated.

Surgery can be used for reconstruction to restore form and function following an operation that has left a physical defect, e.g. following mastectomy. Such procedures can have positive psychological benefits for patients, helping them address issues such as self-image, self-esteem and sexuality.

Palliative procedures

Surgery can still offer palliation for some patients and should be considered when assessing symptoms and problems in patients with cancer. Examples include the following.

- Permanent venous access using indwelling venous catheters for blood sampling and delivery of chemotherapy.
- Abdominal shunts can be placed to drain ascites.
- Debulking of tumours causing chronic pain due to nerve root compression.
- Insertion of percutaneous endoscopic gastrostomy (PEG) feeding tubes to improve nutritional intake.
- Fixation of pathological fractures in bones.
- Defunctioning stoma for bowel obstruction.
- Relieving obstruction of a conduit, such as biliary, hepatic, ureteric, oesophageal or airway obstructions, with stent insertion.

Table 20.1   Examples of common chemotherapy agents

Class	Example agents	Mode of action
Alkylating agents	**Bifunctional alkylating agents** • Nitrogen mustard • Cyclophosphamide • Ifosfamide • Chlorambucil • Melphalan	Alkylating agents transfer an alkyl group to the purine bases of DNA, which are adenine and guanine. Bifunctional alkylating agents form covalent bonds between two different bases, resulting in interstrand or intrastrand cross-links. This inhibits DNA synthesis and therefore acts during S phase of the cell cycle. Bifunctional agents can act on more than one base and are more cytotoxic
	Monofunctional alkylating agents • Dacarbazine • Temozolomide • Nitrosureas	Monofunctional alkylating agents cannot form cross-links but cause adducts. This inhibits DNA synthesis and therefore acts during S phase of the cell cycle. Monofunctional agents are more mutagenic and carcinogenic than bifunctional agents
Intercalating agents	**Platinum compounds** • Cisplatin • Carboplatin • Oxaliplatin	Platinum agents intercalate and disrupt the steric integrity of the DNA double helix but also form intrastrand links similar to those formed by alkylating agents
	Anthracyclines • Doxorubicin • Daunorubicin • Epirubicin **Anthraquinones** • Mitoxantrone	Anthracyclines intercalate into the DNA major groove between base pairs of the DNA double helix. This action is non-covalent and therefore not base specific. This disrupts the steric integrity of the DNA double helix and blocks DNA replication. The main target for these agents is the enzyme topoisomerase II
Topoisomerase I/II inhibitors	**Topoisomerase I inhibitors** • Topotecan • Irinotecan **Topoisomerase II inhibitors** • Etoposide • Teniposide	Topoisomerase enzymes prevent DNA strands from becoming tangled by cutting DNA and allowing it to wind or unwind. Topoisomerase I breaks single-strand DNA and relieves torsion, and inhibitors act in S phase and prevent the re-ligation step of the nicking-closing reaction, trapping topoisomerase I in a covalent complex with DNA. Topoisomerase II breaks both strands of DNA and allows the other strand to pass through and re-ligate
Antimetabolites	**Antifolates** • Methotrexate • Raltitrexed **Pyrimidine analogues** • 5-fluorouracil • Gemcitabine • Cytosine arabinoside **Purine analogues** • 6-mercaptopurine • 6-thioguanine	Antimetabolites are structurally related to natural compounds and inhibit the metabolism of compounds necessary for DNA, RNA, or protein synthesis. Most of these agents have activity during S phase
Tubulin binders	**Vinca alkaloids** • Vincristine • Vinblastine • Vindesine • Vinorelbine **Taxanes** • Paclitaxel • Docetaxel	The vinca alkaloids bind to the tubulin dimer and prevent the assembly of microtubule filaments and therefore interfere with function of the mitotic spindle and prevent cell division during the M phase of the cell cycle. The taxanes bind to tubulin as a polymerised molecule and prevent disassembly back into the dimeric form. They act during the M phase of the cell cycle
Antibodies	Rituximab (CD20) Bevacizumab (VEGF) Trastuzamab (HER2 receptor)	Monoclonal antibodies bind to cell surface proteins expressed in the target tissue. High-affinity binding prevents the normal ligand from attaching and therefore inhibits the normal activation of the receptor. This diminishes the intracellular signal that drives cellular processes such as angiogenesis or cell growth
Kinase inhibitors	Imatinib (BcrAbl, C-Kit) Erlotinib (EGF receptor) Lapatinib (HER2 and EGF receptors)	Kinase inhibitors are small molecules that bind to intracellular domains of a cell-surface receptor and prevent activation of the intracellular signals that drive cellular processes

An introduction to chemotherapy

The origins of chemotherapy lie in the use of biological warfare during the First World War, in the form of mustard gas in 1917. This caused blistering of the skin, conjunctivitis and after about 4 days victims developed myelosuppression. In 1944, the first patient was treated using nitrogen mustard for a lymphoma and achieved a temporary remission but later died of bone marrow failure.

Chemotherapy involves the use of pharmacological agents to kill tumour cells. It can be effective in treating both primary tumours and metastatic spread. Chemotherapy agents act at different stages of the cell cycle and exert their effects primarily by three mechanisms:
- altering the chemistry of nucleic acids;
- interfering with DNA or RNA synthesis;
- disrupting mechanisms of cell division.

Most of the common agents act in a non-selective manner, not only damaging cancer cells but also affecting normal dividing cells such as hair follicles, bone marrow and gastrointestinal mucosa. This produces side effects that limit the dose that can be administered and the recovery time before the next dose can be given. The adverse effects of treatment are discussed in Chapter 22.

Most chemotherapy is given as a combination of drugs administered intravenously on an intermittent basis. An individual cycle is repeated every 21–28 days and a course of treatment typically comprises six cycles of chemotherapy. Malignant cells have less capacity for repair than normal cells and intermittent dosing exploits the fact that tumour cells recover from cytotoxic damage more slowly than normal cell populations. Each sequential treatment cycle aims to deplete tumour cells, while breaks between cycles give normal stem cells time to recover.

Chemotherapy drug dose is usually calculated from the surface area of the patient (based on height and weight). The goals and approach to treatment are outlined in Chapter 18.

Pharmacodynamics is the study of the effects that the drugs have on the body, and dose-limiting toxicity can be used to determine the maximum dose possible in an individual patient. Pharmacokinetics is the study of the effects that the body has on the drugs and can be modified by renal and hepatic function, in addition to metabolism and clearance of the drug from the circulation. Careful monitoring of the patient's biochemistry, renal, liver and bone marrow function is essential during chemotherapy treatment.

Although very effective, chemotherapy is a highly toxic treatment with the potential for life-threatening side effects. It therefore requires supervision from specialists, and patients should have careful assessment prior to commencement of treatment and prior to each cycle. Patient fitness is a reliable predictor of tolerance to treatment; those who are less fit will tolerate chemotherapy less well and will have an increased risk of adverse effects. For this reason, clinicians will carefully assess the patient's performance status using defined scale such as the ECOG and Karnovsky scores (see Chapter 2). Performance status is therefore essential for determining patient suitability for chemotherapy and appropriate dosing of treatments.

Growth fractions and doubling time

Growth fraction is the percentage of cells in a tumour mass that are actively dividing. It may vary from more than 50% in rapidly growing cancers such as Burkitt's lymphoma (doubling time as short as 24 hours) to immeasurable in some adenocarcinomas (which may have a doubling time of up to 200 days).

Chemotherapy agents can be divided into those that are cell cycle independent and those that are cell cycle dependent. The latter can be further subdivided into phase-non-specific, which are equally effective against cells in all phases of the cell cycle except G_0, and phase-specific, which are only active against cells in one phase of the cell cycle. These features can be used to design drug regimen combinations and schedules that take advantage of individual drug characteristics.

The normal process of tissue renewal (e.g. bone marrow, GI mucosa, skin) involves both actively proliferating and quiescent stem cells. The quiescent or resting fraction, those cells in G_0 phase of the cell cycle that are not actively dividing, is important because most anticancer agents are not active against these cells.

A single clonogenic malignant cell is capable of multiplying and ultimately killing the host. This implies that cure depends on total cell eradication of all malignant cells, but there is evidence that in some cancers, there is a host response that may augment chemotherapeutic cell kill.

Tumour growth

The simplest model of tumour growth is that it is exponential, which is true for microscopic lesions with fewer than 10^9 tumour cells. The growth curve of a clinically palpable cancer follows a Gompertzian function, where the rate of growth slows as the tumour increases in size, due to limits imposed by the tumour microenvironment. Larger-volume cancers have smaller growth fractions and thus may be inherently less sensitive to phase-specific agents. Small or micrometastases might be more sensitive to chemotherapy, giving a rationale for adjuvant chemotherapy.

For most chemotherapy agents there is a steep dose response, with greater cell kill demonstrated at higher drug doses. This is true for many experimental models but is more difficult to demonstrate clearly in clinical trials. Moreover, there are other factors that influence cell kill, such as dose intensity or density.

Drug resistance

Resistance may be innate or acquired during treatment. The larger the tumour mass or the more doublings that occur before drug treatment, the more likely it is that there are drug-resistant cells present. Multi-drug resistance has been observed in tumour cells after exposure to a single drug, which can also be resistant to other agents but usually not alkylating agents or antimetabolites. Multidrug resistance is associated with an increased expression of a membrane protein called p-glycoprotein. This functions as an active pump, transporting toxic alkaloids out of the cells. Anticancer drugs are often combined in order to minimise the development of resistance.

Class of chemotherapy agents

The common chemotherapy agents and their mechanism of action are outlined in Table 20.1. They are classified according to their chemical properties and mechanism of action.

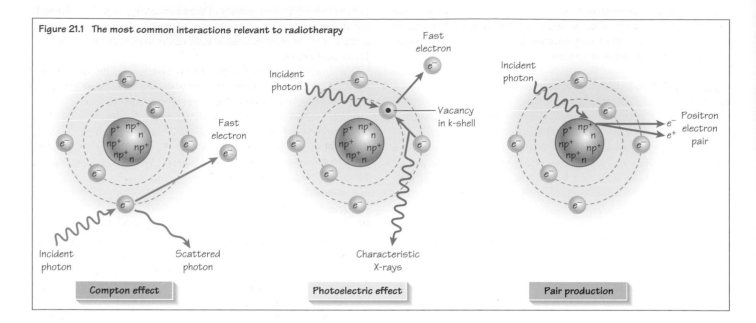

Figure 21.1 The most common interactions relevant to radiotherapy

How radiotherapy works

Radiotherapy is the use of ionising radiation for the treatment of malignant disease. The high-energy electromagnetic waves have sufficient energy to displace an orbital electron from an atom and thus create free radicals. The radiation can be in electromagnetic form such as high-energy photons, or in particulate form such as an electron, a proton, a neutron, or an alpha particle.

The delivery of energy to tissues results in damage to DNA and this diminishes or eradicates the cell's ability to replicate indefinitely. DNA damage caused by free radicals includes damage to nucleotide bases and the carbohydrate backbone, as well as cross-linkage between strands, and single and double strand breaks. Early reactions that occur in tissues that divide rapidly are seen during the course of radiotherapy and are usually reversible. The late effects of radiation are not immediate and may occur many months or even years after the radiation therapy, and are expressed when the cells attempt mitosis and fail. Such effects are less likely to be reversible. This accounts for the apparent delay in tumour response and the timing of radiation reactions in normal tissue.

Malignant cells generally do not have the ability to repair radiation damage and this differentiates them from normal cells. Cells that remain after radiation treatment have access to a greater relative blood supply in addition to other biological factors within the microenvironment of the tumour, such as cytokines or growth factors, and this can lead to cellular repopulation.

Fundamentally, radiation therapy requires oxygen in the target tissues to generate free radicals, which in turn damages the DNA of the tumour cells. Therefore, relative tissue hypoxia will reduce the killing effect of the radiotherapy. Low levels of haemoglobin can further reduce the effect of radiation treatment for the same reason.

High-energy photons

This is the most common form of radiation used in practice, where photons are released from the nucleus of a radioactive atom and are known as gamma rays. When photons are created in a linear accelerator, they are known as X-rays. Therefore, the only difference between the two terms is the origin of the photon.

Photoelectric effect

Incoming photons collide with a tightly bound electron in the target tissue and transfer the majority of their energy to the electron and cease to exist. The electrons begin to ionise the surrounding molecules and this interaction depends on the energy level of the incoming photons, as well as the atomic number of the target tissue. For example, the atomic number of bone is 60% higher than that of soft tissue and therefore bone is seen with more contrast and detail than soft tissue. The energy range in which the photoelectric effect predominates in tissue is about 10–25 keV.

Compton effect

A photon collides with an electron that is not tightly bound to the atom, resulting in both the photon and electron being scattered. The photon can continue to have additional interactions at a lower energy, while the electron can ionise with the energy donated by the photon. The probability of such an interaction is inversely proportional to the energy of the incoming photon and is independent of the atomic number of the material. This effect is the most common interaction occurring in radiotherapy practice, as most radiation treatments are performed at energy levels of about 6–20 MeV.

Pair production

In pair production, a photon interacts with the nucleus of an atom instead of an orbital electron. The photon donates its energy to the nucleus and creates a pair of positively and negatively charged electrons. The positive electron (positron) ionises until it combines with a free electron and generates two photons, which scatter in opposite directions. The probability of pair production is proportional to the logarithm of the energy of the incoming photon and is dependent on the atomic number of the target material. The energy range in which pair production dominates is 25 MeV.

Types of radiation treatment

Electron beams

With high-energy linear accelerators, electron therapy can treat superficial tumours up to a depth of 5 cm. Electron depth dose characteristics are unique in that they produce a high skin dose but exhibit a fall-off after only a few centimetres. Electron absorption in human tissue is influenced by the presence of air cavities and bone, with increased delivered dose when the beam passes through an air space and reduced dose when the beam passes through bone.

Electrons are used for the treatment of skin lesions (e.g. basal cell carcinomas) or to boost the dose to areas pretreated with photons.

Brachytherapy

Brachytherapy is the local treatment of a tumour where the radiation source is in contact with the tumour. The dose distribution is dependent on the inverse square law because the source is usually within the tumour volume and therefore correct placement of the radiation source is crucial. In the past, radium was used as a source, but has been replaced with caesium (Cs), gold (Au) and iridium (Ir), which have shorter half-lives and can be shielded more easily because of their lower energies.

Brachytherapy is used in cancer of the oral cavity, oropharynx and sarcoma. Prostate cancer is probably the most common site treated with brachytherapy in addition to gynaecologic cancers (e.g. cervix).

Conformal radiation therapy

This is a geometric shaping of the radiation beam that conforms with the shape of the tumour from the perspective of the beam source. Conformal therapy requires CT simulation, and the oncologist outlines the tumour volume and draws an appropriate margin from 1 to 2 cm around the tumour. These fields conform closely to the shape of the tumour and thus shield more critical structures than do normal blocks. The tolerance of this planning allows for set-up errors of a few millimetres each day and patients are immobilised by using casts that constrain the movement of the relevant part of the patient's body.

As the treatment volume is more closely matched to the target tumour volume, the delivered dose can be increased as there will be reduced toxicity in the surrounding normal tissues. The intensity of the beam remains constant.

Intensity-modulated radiation therapy (IMRT)

An extension of conformal therapy, this allows for shaping of the radiation beam or modulation of the beam intensity while the treatment is delivered. This is an important improvement, especially when the target is not well separated from normal tissues, and allows for a uniform dose distribution around the tumour. This is achieved by either modulating the intensity of the beam during its journey through the linear accelerator or by the use of multileaf collimators, which consist of 80 or more individual collimators located at the head of the linear accelerator.

The result is a uniform dose distribution around the tumour and minimal dose to the surrounding normal tissues, often below tolerance levels, which reduces the risk of toxicity to normal tissues.

IMRT is therefore considered where the target tumour is in close proximity to important normal structures. For example, head and neck tumours, where the salivary glands can be avoided; or for prostate cancer, to reduce toxicity to nearby structures, allowing doses to be increased significantly without increasing the complication rate.

Proton therapy

Protons are a form of particulate radiation where the particle is stable with a charge of +1 and, together with the neutron, makes up the atomic nucleus. Protons can be delivered in the same manner as photons and electrons, where the kinetic energy causes electrons to be displaced from molecules in the target tissue. The biological effect of protons is similar to that of megavoltage photons, where the free radicals produced cause DNA damage. However, in contrast to photons, the dose deposited by protons remains relatively constant as they travel through the normal tissues proximal to the target.

At the end of the path of the protons, they slow down and eventually stop. As they slow and stop, their biological effectiveness increases sharply and this increase in dose is called the Bragg peak. The size of the Bragg peak is usually smaller than the tumour and this dose fall-off is sharp enough that the normal tissues distal to the tumour receive a negligible dose of radiation. This is particularly useful where the tumour is adjacent to sensitive tissue such as the CNS or other important normal structures.

Stereotactic radiosurgery

This is a three-dimensional technique that delivers the radiation dose in a single treatment fraction. A linear accelerator delivers a high dose of radiation to a small volume, usually about 3 cm in diameter, using several stationary beams or multiple arc rotations to concentrate the radiation dose at the site of the tumour while sparing the surrounding normal tissue.

Stereotactic radiosurgery has been used to treat intracranial arteriovenous malformations and although surgical excision is the treatment of choice, stereotactic radiosurgery has become a viable option for inoperable malformations.

This stereotactic approach is used for treating brain tumours, either with a dedicated cobalt unit (Gamma knife) or a linear accelerator-based system.

Figure 22.1 Clinical features of adverse effects of treatment

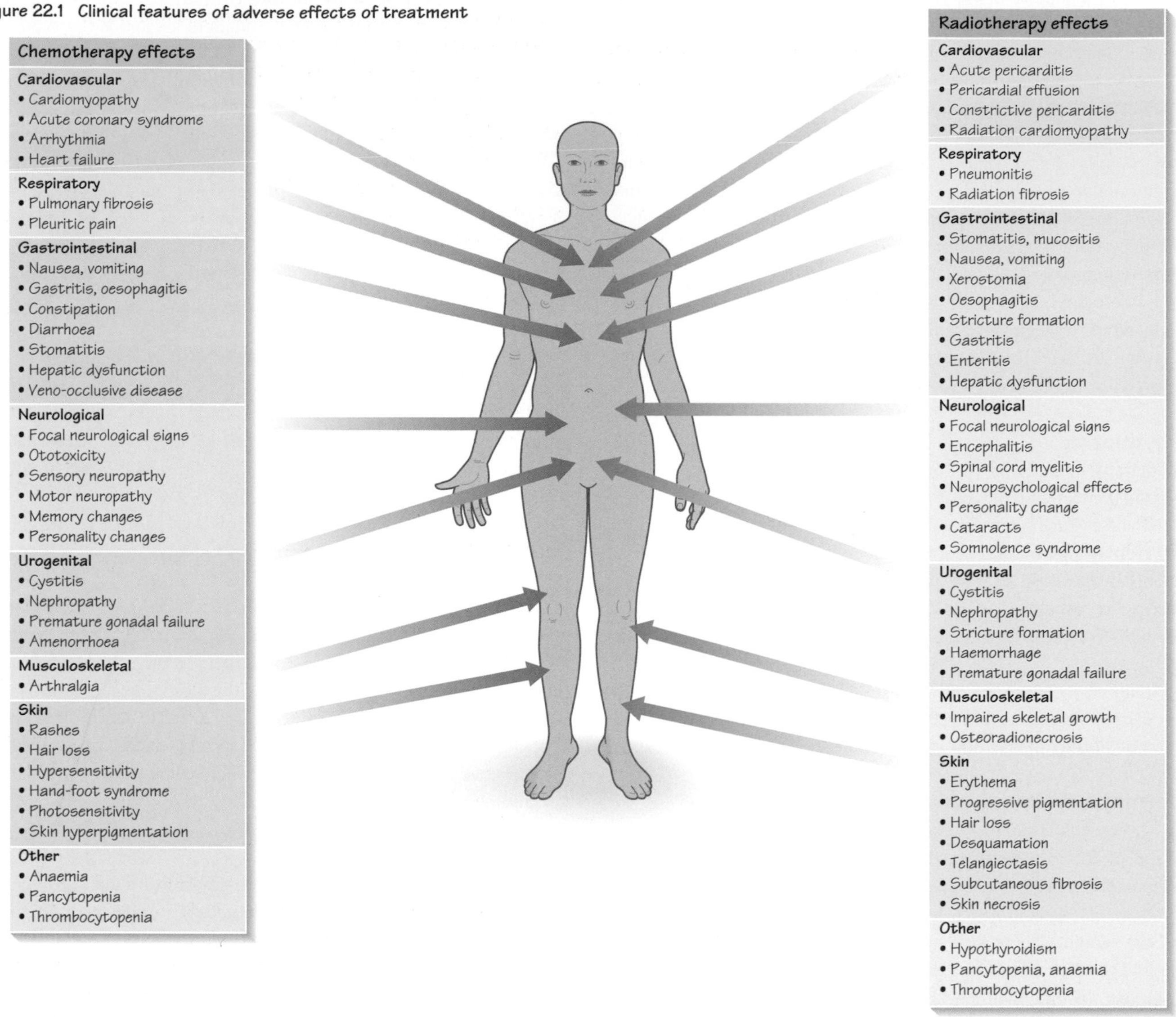

Chemotherapy effects

Cardiovascular
- Cardiomyopathy
- Acute coronary syndrome
- Arrhythmia
- Heart failure

Respiratory
- Pulmonary fibrosis
- Pleuritic pain

Gastrointestinal
- Nausea, vomiting
- Gastritis, oesophagitis
- Constipation
- Diarrhoea
- Stomatitis
- Hepatic dysfunction
- Veno-occlusive disease

Neurological
- Focal neurological signs
- Ototoxicity
- Sensory neuropathy
- Motor neuropathy
- Memory changes
- Personality changes

Urogenital
- Cystitis
- Nephropathy
- Premature gonadal failure
- Amenorrhoea

Musculoskeletal
- Arthralgia

Skin
- Rashes
- Hair loss
- Hypersensitivity
- Hand-foot syndrome
- Photosensitivity
- Skin hyperpigmentation

Other
- Anaemia
- Pancytopenia
- Thrombocytopenia

Radiotherapy effects

Cardiovascular
- Acute pericarditis
- Pericardial effusion
- Constrictive pericarditis
- Radiation cardiomyopathy

Respiratory
- Pneumonitis
- Radiation fibrosis

Gastrointestinal
- Stomatitis, mucositis
- Nausea, vomiting
- Xerostomia
- Oesophagitis
- Stricture formation
- Gastritis
- Enteritis
- Hepatic dysfunction

Neurological
- Focal neurological signs
- Encephalitis
- Spinal cord myelitis
- Neuropsychological effects
- Personality change
- Cataracts
- Somnolence syndrome

Urogenital
- Cystitis
- Nephropathy
- Stricture formation
- Haemorrhage
- Premature gonadal failure

Musculoskeletal
- Impaired skeletal growth
- Osteoradionecrosis

Skin
- Erythema
- Progressive pigmentation
- Hair loss
- Desquamation
- Telangiectasis
- Subcutaneous fibrosis
- Skin necrosis

Other
- Hypothyroidism
- Pancytopenia, anaemia
- Thrombocytopenia

Treatment toxicity

The adverse effects of radiotherapy and chemotherapy are classified in temporal groupings depending on the time of onset. **Early effects** are seen during treatment or within the first few weeks after its completion. Reactions are common, and can be very significant and symptomatic. Most common chemotherapy effects are early and although they resolve there can be long-term residual damage. **Intermediate effects** occur several weeks to months after the completion of treatment, and **late effects** are usually rare and are encountered many months to years after treatment. Functional impairments may take a very long time to become apparent; an example is memory problems in children who have received cranial irradiation. The development of a secondary malignancy is more common following radiotherapy.

Extravasation injury

During administration a drug can leak into the surrounding subcutaneous tissue. The consequences are local inflammatory reactions at the infusion site. There is no permanent damage if the drug is an irritant substance. Extravasation of vesicant agents has the potential to cause severe or irreversible tissue injury and necrosis (anthracyclines, vinca alkaloids). In some cases the tissue necrosis can require skin grafting and has the potential for extensive disfigurement. If extravasation is suspected, IV therapy should be stopped immediately and the site massaged to remove any obvious liquid from the site. Local protocol should then be followed, with early involvement of the plastic surgery team. Patency of intravenous access should be tested regularly with patients educated to report any pain or odd sensations.

Specific toxicities

Alopecia usually occurs 3–6 weeks after the first dose of some chemotherapeutic agents, producing significant psychological impact.

Cardiac toxicity can be in the form of arrhythmia (paclitaxel), acute pericarditis (radiotherapy), pericardial effusion and cardiomyopathy (anthracyclines and radiotherapy).

Gastrointestinal tract toxicity includes: stomatitis (doxorubicin, 5-fluorouracil), ulceration, diarrhoea (irinotecan, topotecan, paclitaxel), constipation (carboplatin), enteritis (5-fluorouracil, actinomycin-D, cisplatin, methotrexate, hydroxyurea, procarbazine), proctocolitis (radiotherapy) and oesophagitis (doxorubicin, cyclophosphamide).

Hepatic toxicity is due to direct effects on the hepatocytes and can result in cholestasis (6-mercaptopurine), acute liver necrosis (high-dose methotrexate, asparaginase, mithramycin), hepatic fibrosis (chronic low-dose methotrexate) and veno-occlusive disease (high-dose chemotherapy with autologous stem-cell rescue).

Musculoskeletal toxicity can produce arthralgia (paclitaxel) and osteoradionecrosis, a hypovascular, hypocellular dissolution of bone secondary to radiotherapy. Dental extractions performed after radiotherapy to the head and neck can initiate osteoradionecrosis. Impairment of skeletal growth can occur following radiotherapy to growing bone end plates in children.

Myelosuppression with neutropenia (increasing the risk of infection), thrombocytopenia (risk of bruising) and anaemia causing tiredness and lethargy.

Nausea and vomiting is covered in Chapter 24.

Nephrotoxicity most commonly results from chemotherapy (carboplatin, cisplatin, methotrexate, mitomycin-C), producing electrolyte disturbance and reduced glomerular filtration rate (GFR). Radiotherapy can reduce the GFR but this is rarely symptomatic.

Nervous system toxicity as peripheral sensory and motor neuropathy (cisplatin, vincristine), cerebellar degeneration (5-fluorouracil/high-dose arabinoside), encephalopathy (ifosfamide, asparaginase), myelopathy (intrathecal methotrexate, spinal cord radiotherapy), or reduced intelligence quotient (IQ) (craniospinal radiotherapy for childhood leukaemia). Early complications of radiotherapy (first 3–4 months) are due to reversible damage to myelin-producing oligodendrocytes that recover spontaneously after 3–6 months. It causes somnolence or exacerbation of existing symptoms in the brain and Lhermitte's sign (shooting numbness or paraesthesia precipitated by neck flexion) in the cord. Late radiotherapy effects include irreversible necrosis due to vessel damage, which can mimic disease recurrence. It is radiation dose related and occurs in up to 15% of patients, with the highest frequency in children receiving concurrent chemotherapy. PET imaging may help distinguish radionecrosis and relapse.

Pulmonary toxicity can be irreversible and produce significant impact in the form of fibrosis (bleomycin, busulphan, methotrexate, mitomycin C, BCNU). Radiotherapy can produce pneumonitis 1–3 months after the completion of therapy, which can be lethal if both lungs are involved. Acute symptoms include low-grade fever, congestion, cough, dyspnoea, pleuritic chest pain and haemoptysis. Chest X-ray and CT imaging show a diffuse infiltrate corresponding to the radiation field. Pulmonary fibrosis develops insidiously in the previously irradiated field and stabilises after 1–2 years, with most patients being asymptomatic.

Reproductive system toxicity results from direct effects of radiotherapy or chemotherapy on intact ovaries or testes. Following chemotherapy (or high-dose radiotherapy), premenopausal women can develop ovarian suppression with menopausal symptoms and infertility, which can take 18 months to fully recover. Testicular dysfunction with hormonal changes may result from chemotherapy.

Skin toxicity can manifest as rashes due to hypersensitivity (carboplatin, paclitaxel), palmar-plantar erythrodysaesthesia (5-fluorouracil, capcitabine, liposomal doxorubicin) and acute skin reactions 7–10 days after radiotherapy, with erythema, progressive pigmentation, epilation and desquamation as the dose increases. Late effects many weeks following radiotherapy include scaling, atrophy, telangiectasis, subcutaneous fibrosis and necrosis.

Teratogenesis can result with some agents and therefore condoms should be used during intercourse for the first 48 hours after chemotherapy to protect a partner from exposure to any drug that may be present in semen or vaginal fluid.

Urothelial toxicity can be acute and manifest as cystitis and haemorrhage (radiation, ifosfamide). Late effects of radiotherapy occur after a median of 13–20 months with decreased bladder capacity, haematuria from telangiectasis, chronic irritation or obstructive symptoms, and fistulas. Urethral strictures occur more frequently when there is a history of a prior transurethral resection of the prostate.

Late adverse effects

The late toxicities of treatment for cancer are particularly important for patients where the treatment is given with curative intent and more patients are living longer. Late effects of multimodality therapy on the developing child are substantial, and the late sequelae cause considerable morbidity in this group of patients where the long-term survival rates are high. Radiotherapy can retard bone and cartilage growth, impair intellect and cognitive function, and cause dysfunction of the hypothalamus and thyroid glands. Late consequences of chemotherapy include heart failure due to cardiotoxicity, pulmonary fibrosis, nephrotoxicity and neurotoxicity.

Premature gonadal failure can result from chemotherapy or radiotherapy and leave a patient subfertile. Patients should be made aware of this before initiating treatment as it may be possible to store sperm for male patients before treatment starts and this should always be offered if practical. Oligospermia occurs after very low doses of radiotherapy and can therefore be precipitated by exposure to scattered radiotherapy from other treatment sites, as well as by total-body irradiation used as a conditioning regimen for bone marrow transplantation. Sterility develops at higher radiotherapy doses but erectile dysfunction is seen in patients receiving high radiotherapy doses to the pelvis, as in prostate cancer. Additional social or psychological support may be required to deal with this issue.

Second malignancies may be induced by anticancer treatment and occur at greatest frequency following chemoradiation. Secondary acute leukaemia (mostly AML) can occur 1–2 years after treatment with topoisomerase II inhibitors with abnormalities of chromosome 11q23, or can occur 2–5 years after treatment with alkylating agents with abnormalities of chromosome 5q. The most common second malignancy within a radiation field is osteosarcoma, but others include soft tissue sarcoma and leukaemia.

Management of nausea

Figure 23.1 Neural pathways in vomiting

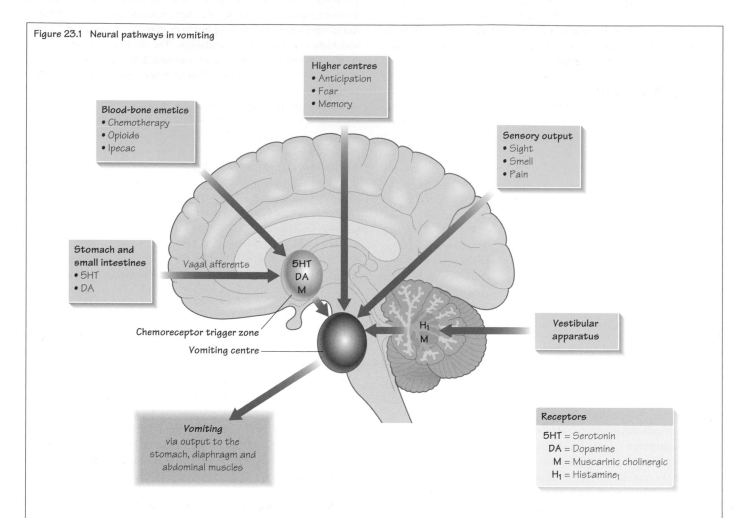

Table 23.1 Types of nausea and vomiting in patients with cancer

Classification	Timescale	Causative factors	Treatment approach
Acute	<24 hours after chemotherapy	Many chemotherapy drugs will cause chemotherapy-induced nausea and vomiting (CINV)	Dexamethasone Metoclopramide Ondansetron
Delayed (or late)	>24 hours after chemotherapy	Many chemotherapy drugs, particularly cisplatin, cyclophosphamide, dacarbazine, methotrexate, mitomycin-C	Dexamethasone Ondansetron Aprepitant Treat any associated constipation
Anticipatory	Prior to a new cycle of chemotherapy	Conditioned stimuli such as sights, smells or sounds in the chemotherapy unit; often occurs after 3–4 cycles of treatment	Benzodiazepines Progressive muscle relaxation Hypnotherapy
Chronic	Long-term nausea in advanced cancer	Varied and complex, patient-dependent and usually in patients with advanced disease	Requires a careful assessment of the patient's symptoms and application of anti-emetics best directed at the underlying cause

Nausea and vomiting are common, distressing symptoms that affect many cancer patients (Table 23.1). Patients can develop nutritional complications, dehydration and electrolyte imbalance as a result, which can delay or compromise the delivery of systemic chemotherapy. Despite advances in pharmacological and non-pharmacological treatments, nausea and vomiting remain major apprehensions for patients awaiting their first treatment.

Pathophysiology

Vomiting is controlled by a vomiting centre in the floor of the fourth ventricle of the brain, which receives signals from the chemoreceptor trigger zone (CTZ), hypothalamus, cerebral cortex and the vestibular apparatus. The role of the vomiting centre is to coordinate the complex process of vomiting.

Nausea is an unpleasant sensation accompanied by reduced gastric motility with increased contraction of the duodenum. Peripheral stimuli to the vomiting centre arise from the gut through the autonomic nervous system and the vagal nerve. Other stimuli include visceral stimulation (e.g. stomach after ingestion of exogenous chemical), vestibular stimulation (e.g. vertigo), sensory stimuli (e.g. foul smell), chemical stimuli (e.g. chemotherapy) and impulses from the chemoreceptor trigger zone directly (Figure 23.1).

The CTZ is a highly vascularised area of the brain designed to sample blood and CSF for chemicals that can trigger emesis, particularly following exposure to chemotherapy and opioid analgesia. There is considerable variation among individuals, which accounts for the variability in emetogenicity between different medications and different people.

Oncology practice

Not all cancer patients are affected by nausea and vomiting, but there are common patterns encountered in clinical practice, and a detailed medical history will aid diagnosis of the underlying cause.
- **Iatrogenic:** chemotherapy, opioid analgesia (constipation may contribute), radiotherapy-induced toxicity of the gut, liver or brain.
- **Metabolic disturbances:** hypercalcaemia, hyponatraemia, water imbalance (retention or depletion) or uraemia.
- **Direct tumour effects:** malignant bowel obstruction, liver metastasis, raised intracranial pressure due to CNS metastasis.
- **Psychogenic:** anticipatory nausea, anxiety.

Approach to treatment

Anti-emetic medication is designed to impair the neurochemical initiation of vomiting within the CNS. Most agents act by competitive inhibition of neurotransmitters such as dopamine or serotonin, thus decreasing stimulation to the CTZ and the vomiting centre.

Anti-emetics can be administered orally prior to planned chemotherapy or radiation treatment, with parenteral administration used if the patient begins vomiting. The choice of anti-emetic therapy for chemotherapy-induced nausea and vomiting depends on the emetogenicity of the chemotherapy drug used. For high-risk treatment combination regimens using serotonin antagonists, steroids and a neurokinin-1 (NK-1) receptor antagonist (aprepitant) are used, whereas low-risk treatment may only require metoclopramide treatment.

The mechanism of action of the commonly used anti-emetic medications are described below.

Phenothiazines (e.g. prochlorperazine, prochlorpromazine) act primarily on the CTZ but also have antihistaminic and anticholinergic action. Prochlorperazine is commonly used to prevent nausea associated with low emetogenic chemotherapy or radiation therapy. Administration is usually oral but high-dose IV regimes can be used with highly emetogenic chemotherapy. The most common side effects of all dopaminergic antagonists are sedation and extra-pyramidal symptoms such as dystonia, Parkinsonism, akathisia and tardive dyskinesia.

Antihistamines (e.g. promethazine, cyclizine) act on the vomiting centre directly and are the drugs of choice for motion sickness or vestibular-mediated nausea.

Butyrophenones such as haloperidol have a long half-life and work best in cases of chemical stimulation of the CTZ, particularly opioid-induced nausea and vomiting.

Serotonin antagonists (e.g. ondansetron, granisetron, dolasteron and palonosetron) are commonly used to prevent chemotherapy-induced nausea and vomiting, particularly from highly emetogenic treatments such as cisplatin-containing regimens. It has a superior anti-emetic control to metoclopramide and a lower incidence of side effects such as headache, constipation, dry mouth and fatigue.

Metoclopramide is a substituted benzamide, most effective when given at high dose intravenously for acute vomiting. However, it is commonly used to prevent chemotherapy-induced nausea in low to medium emetogenic treatments. It acts directly on the CTZ and promotes gastrointestinal motility and gastric emptying. Side effects include sedation and extrapyramidal symptoms.

Domperidone does not cross the blood–brain barrier and therefore does not cause the central adverse effects of metoclopramide. It acts as a more selective peripheral dopamine blocker.

Other classes of medications include substance P antagonists, corticosteroids (usually added to other medication), benzodiazepines and olanzapine. These are less commonly used and carry risks of several potentially severe side effects.

Patients with advanced disease

Chronic nausea in patients with advanced cancer is usually multifactorial in origin. Such patients are often taking opioid analgesia, suffer from constipation, can be dehydrated, suffer from poor nutritional intake and metabolic disturbances. They require careful assessment and treatment as they may develop complications such as electrolyte imbalance or acid-base disturbance. Occasionally drug-induced nausea may be alleviated by administering drugs with food or by taking regular anti-emetic medication.

Constipation is a common contributing factor and should be treated aggressively with regular laxative therapy.

For patients unable to take oral medication a subcutaneous infusion and other parenteral routes may be used. The role of serotonin antagonists in chronic nausea is limited.

Patients with intractable nausea should be investigated, as underlying causes such as malignant bowel obstruction, hypercalcaemia, hyponatraemia, uraemia with deteriorating renal function, or brain metastasis may be identified. Treatment of the underlying problem will improve the patient's symptoms.

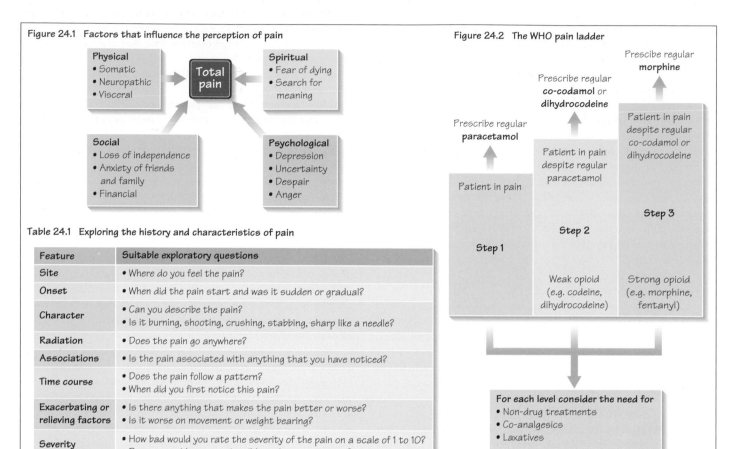

Figure 24.1 Factors that influence the perception of pain

Physical
- Somatic
- Neuropathic
- Visceral

Total pain

Spiritual
- Fear of dying
- Search for meaning

Social
- Loss of independence
- Anxiety of friends and family
- Financial

Psychological
- Depression
- Uncertainty
- Despair
- Anger

Figure 24.2 The WHO pain ladder

Prescribe regular **paracetamol**

Prescribe regular **co-codamol** or **dihydrocodeine**

Prescibe regular **morphine**

Patient in pain — **Step 1**

Patient in pain despite regular paracetamol — **Step 2**

Patient in pain despite regular co-codamol or dihydrocodeine — **Step 3**

Weak opioid (e.g. codeine, dihydrocodeine)

Strong opioid (e.g. morphine, fentanyl)

For each level consider the need for
- Non-drug treatments
- Co-analgesics
- Laxatives

Table 24.1 Exploring the history and characteristics of pain

Feature	Suitable exploratory questions
Site	• Where do you feel the pain?
Onset	• When did the pain start and was it sudden or gradual?
Character	• Can you describe the pain? • Is it burning, shooting, crushing, stabbing, sharp like a needle?
Radiation	• Does the pain go anywhere?
Associations	• Is the pain associated with anything that you have noticed?
Time course	• Does the pain follow a pattern? • When did you first notice this pain?
Exacerbating or relieving factors	• Is there anything that makes the pain better or worse? • Is it worse on movement or weight bearing?
Severity	• How bad would you rate the severity of the pain on a scale of 1 to 10? • Do you consider your pain mild, moderate or severe?
Impact	• Does the pain affect your sleep? • Does the pain stop you doing things? • Does the pain affect your appetite? • Does the pain affect your mood? • Can you do your normal work?
Treatments	• What have you tried for pain relief? • How much pain was taken away by a particular drug?

Table 24.2 Adjuvant therapies used as co-analgesia approaches

Common drug groups	Example drugs	Indications
Anticonvulsants	Carbamazepine	Neuropathic pain, tenesmoid pain
Antidepressants	Amitriptyline	Neuropathic pain, tenesmoid pain
Anti-emetics	Haloperidol, metoclopramide	Opioid-induced nausea, particularly at initiation of therapy
Bisphosphonates	Pamidronate	Bone pain
Corticosteroids	Dexamethasone	Raised intracranial pressure, nerve compression, liver capsular pain, soft tissue infiltration
Muscle relaxants	Baclofen, diazepam	Muscle cramp, spasm, myofacial pain
NSAIDs	Diclofenac, ibuprofen	Bone pain, soft tissue infiltration
Sedation	Midazolam, temazepam, nitrazepam	Sleep disturbance, agitation

Pain is defined as an unpleasant sensory and emotional experience with actual or potential tissue damage. It is highly subjective and therefore open to modification. The idea of total pain (Figure 24.1) should be used when considering its management.

Pain is one of the most feared symptoms of malignant disease, with at least two-thirds of cancer patients suffering significant pain throughout the course of their disease. Patients with cancer can have multiple sites of pain and multiple types of pain, and each requires careful assessment and treatment (Table 24.1).

Pain assessment

Cancer does not always cause pain, but if it does, assessment may be difficult due to complex or multiple sites of involvement. Ensure there is thorough assessment and documentation for each pain, remembering that some pains may change with time, therefore requiring reassessment. It is important to determine the patient's ideas, concerns and expectations, ensuring they have realistic expectations of treatment. Explore their social, psychological and spiritual issues regarding their pain and remember that these are significant to how they will perceive and manage their discomfort. Physical examination may help establish a cause, and imaging may be required.

Pain is multifactorial, either directly related to the malignancy or indirectly due to systemic complication (e.g. due to cachexia or pressure sores), or due to pre-existing co-morbidities.

Somatic pain is transmitted via the spinothalamic tract. This decussates at the level of the spinal cord, transmitting to the cortex via the thalamus, giving intensity and topographical location of the stimuli. It is commonly described as crushing, tearing and throbbing, and is usually well localised.

Neuropathic pain can arise from damage to nerves, either peripherally or centrally, due to compression, ischaemia, haemorrhage, chemicals, or transection. Damaged neurones can discharge spontaneously and can recruit healthy neurones due to cross-talk, exaggerating the pain. Persistent hyperexcitation can result in hyperalgesia and allodynia. Neuropathic pain is described as burning, shooting, stabbing, or 'pins and needles'.

Inflammatory pain results from peripheral or central mediators of inflammation. Cytokines (IL-1, IL-6, TNFα) create feedback loops, which sensitise primary afferent nerves causing peripheral hyperalgesia. These can be inhibited peripherally via opioid receptors or COX pathways.

Visceral pain can be differentiated from somatic pain by its diffuse, poorly localised nature. It is stimulated by chemical insult, ischaemia, inflammation, or compression or distension of organs. Serotonin (5-HT) is a key transmitter both centrally and peripherally.

Treatment

The World Health Organization (WHO) has produced an analgesic pain ladder guiding the choice of analgesic according to severity of pain (Figure 24.2). At each level, the patient should be assessed for need of co-analgesics, laxatives and adjuvants, with examples outlined in Table 24.2. Other non-drug approaches include the following.
- **Interventional methods** such as spinal analgesia, nerve blockade, radiotherapy, orthopaedic or spinal surgical stabilisation.

- **Non-interventional measures** such as transcutaneous electrical nerve stimulation (TENS), acupuncture, massage, hydrotherapy and complementary therapies.
- **Rehabilitative support** with physiotherapy or occupational therapy.
- **Behavioural techniques** such as relaxation training, hypnosis and music therapy can be useful for some patients particularly those who have lost self-control.

Opioid analgesia

Healthcare professionals and patients are sometimes apprehensive about using strong opioid analgesia. When titrated appropriately against moderate or severe pain, addiction is very rare and side effects manageable. Some forms of pain may be opioid resistant and patients may be sedated without achieving analgesia. If increasing doses fail to control the pain this should be recognised and specialist advice sought from palliative or acute pain teams.

Mild pain is treated with paracetamol or NSAIDs such as aspirin, ibuprofen, or diclofenac.

Moderate pain requires a weak opioid such as codeine or dihydrocodeine, but constipation is often a problem and requires the concomitant use of regular laxatives.

Severe pain requires a strong opioid such as morphine, fentanyl, oxycodone, methadone, hydromorphone, or diamorphine. Drugs should be prescribed for regular administration rather than ad hoc and caution should be used in patients with renal impairment who may accumulate the drug, particularly if using a long-acting preparation. Regular co-analgesics such as paracetamol should be prescribed at the same time to reduce the dose of opioids, and patients should be educated about the use of breakthrough doses of their drugs. Patients who cannot tolerate oral medication due to swallowing difficulties can be considered for alternative routes, such as transdermal, rectal and subcutaneous.

Side effects

Long-term consequences such as tolerance, dependence, hyperalgesia and suppression of the hypothalamic pituitary axis should be recognised along with the following more common side effects.

Constipation is the most common and can persist throughout treatment, thus all patients should receive concomitant laxatives.

Nausea and vomiting can be seen at initiation of opioid treatment, but patients usually become tolerant within a week and should receive prophylactic haloperidol or metoclopramide in this period.

Sedation is common in the first few days of treatment or if the dose is too generous. Patients receiving radiotherapy or other treatment of the underlying cancer can see their pain improve and hence require reduced doses of analgesia.

Opioid toxicity can produce drowsiness, myoclonic jerks, pinpoint pupils (miosis), hallucinations, confusion and respiratory depression. If toxicity occurs, the renal function and dosing schedule should be reviewed carefully. Consider reducing the dose or switching to an alternative opioid.

Other adverse effects include dry mouth, sweating, itching and urinary retention.

Careful continuing assessment of requirements is an integral part of cancer pain management.

25 Clinical trials in cancer patients

Table 25.1 Purpose and typical endpoints of anticancer therapy clinical trials

Study type	Purpose of study	Research approach	Typical trial endpoints
Phase I	• Determine MTD • Observe patterns of toxicity • Pharmacokinetics • Recommend dose for phase II evaluation	• Dose often starts at one-tenth the lethal dose in the most sensitive species • Pre-planned dose escalation is made • if no acute toxicity is seen in a cohort of 3–6 patients • If there is acute toxicity in 33% of patients, three more are treated at the same level • If no further dose-limiting toxicity (DLT) is seen, the dose level is escalated for the next cohort • If the incidence of DLT is seen in >33% of patients at a given level, then dose escalation stops • The phase II recommended dose often is taken as the highest dose for which the incidence of DLT is less than 33%	• Evaluation of toxicity • Response rate
Phase II	• Determine efficacy and safety • Measure toxicity • Correlation with biological or molecular parameters	• Dose is informed by the phase I evaluation • Investigators should determine a target activity level of interest • A variety of statistical accrual plans and sample size methods have been developed but a two-stage design is often used • Patients are entered into the first stage and if fewer than predicted responses are obtained, accrual terminates and the drug is rejected as being of little interest • Otherwise, accrual continues to a second stage and at the end, the drug is rejected if the observed response rate is less than predicted as determined by the design employed	• Disease-free survival • Progression-free survival • Evaluation of toxicity • Response rates • Quality of life
Phase III	• Direct comparison of study arm against a standard control • Determine efficacy and safety • Measure toxicity • Correlation with biological or molecular parameters • Economic comparison	• The protocol for a phase III trial should specify the number of patients to be accrued, duration of follow-up after study closure and time points when analysis will be performed • Sample size planning is based on the assumption that at the conclusion of the follow-up period, a statistical significance test will be performed comparing the experimental treatment to the control treatment with regard to a single primary end point • A statistical significance level of 0.05 means that if there is no true difference in treatment effectiveness, the probability of obtaining a difference in outcomes as extreme as that observed in the data is 0.05. The significance level does not represent the probability that the null hypothesis is true, more a probability that an observed difference is true • With few patients in the trial, the difference in observed outcomes must be extreme in order to obtain statistical significance. Consequently, the probability of obtaining a statistically significant result may be low even when a substantial true difference in effectiveness exists • The probability of obtaining a statistically significant result when the treatments differ in effectiveness is called the power of the trial. The power depends critically, however, on the size of the true difference in effectiveness of the two treatments. • As the sample size and extent of follow-up increases, the power increases. Generally, the study design is with a power of either 0.80 or 0.90 when the true difference in effectiveness is the smallest size that is considered medically important to detect • One of the important principles in the analysis of phase III trials is the intention-to-treat principle. This indicates that all randomised patients should be included in the primary analysis of the trial	• Disease-free survival • Progression-free survival • Overall survival • Response rates • Evaluation of toxicity (early and late) • Quality of life • Economics

Asking a research question

Clinical trials are experiments using patients to determine the value of a treatment or intervention. There are two key components to the experimental approach: objective results rather than plausible reasoning to support conclusions, and that the trials are prospectively planned and conducted under controlled conditions in order to provide definitive answers to well-defined questions. All clinical trials involving patients should be conducted under the regulations for Good Clinical Practice and by suitably trained investigators.

Observational studies

In observational studies, the investigators are passive rapporteurs and the treatment assignment, investigations and follow-up procedures are out of the control of the investigators and conducted with no considerations about the validity of the subsequent attempt at comparison. Such studies are a weak basis for causal inferences about relationships between the treatments administered and the outcomes observed. Observational studies are generally the only feasible approach for epidemiological assessment of disease aetiology. Acute observations in poorly structured therapeutic settings can lead to the development of valuable ideas that can be tested in the laboratory or in clinical trials. Observational studies are rarely satisfactory alternatives to clinical trials.

Phase I clinical trials

The objectives of a phase I trial are to determine the maximum tolerated dose (MTD) of drug for a given schedule and route of delivery, the pattern of adverse effects and toxicity, and to measure the antitumour activity. Pharmacokinetic studies are often conducted in parallel, and at the end a recommended dose for phase II evaluation is determined. Patients considered for such cancer studies are those who have a good performance status as well as adequate organ function and for whom there is no effective alternative treatment available.

Phase II clinical trials

A phase II study is designed to explore whether the drug works in a variety of tumour types, but usually in the patient group in which it is most likely to show a favourable effect. Patient selection is important and only those with good performance status and adequate organ function should be considered. A phase II trial can be of a new agent or an existing drug given at a different dose, schedule or sequence with other drugs. The main objective is to determine whether the drug or combination has activity, and objective response rate is the most common endpoint for measurement. The response to a treatment is not a direct measure of patient benefit, as treatment that causes a partial response is not necessarily beneficial to the patient. Furthermore, it cannot be concluded that a treatment extends survival even if responders live longer than non-responders. To conclude that there are survival gains, it must be demonstrated that the treated group as a whole lives longer than an appropriate matched control group (i.e. a phase III). Phase II trials do not have such an internal control, hence conclusions about survival may not be valid.

The conclusions of phase II trials of combinations are comparative and should be made against a prognostically similar group of patients given standard treatment. Such historical control comparisons are not sufficiently reliable and this requires a phase III trial to evaluate. Drugs should not progress beyond phase II evaluation if no significant effectiveness is observed, toxicity is seen below the active drug level, there are formulation difficulties, or if there is inadequate testing.

Phase III clinical trials

A phase I trial informs the dose of the drug that can be given and phase II gives evidence of whether it works. If the treatment looks promising the next question is whether it works better than that currently available. To answer this requires a prospective, randomised controlled phase III clinical trial. Some phase III trials lack focus and do not ask important questions, and sometimes the most important studies are the most difficult to conduct. For example, a study might involve withholding an established treatment, transferring the management responsibility for a patient across specialties, standardising a procedure among clinicians who believe that their way is best, and sharing recognition with a large group of collaborators.

Phase III trials attempt to provide guidance to practising clinicians to inform treatment decisions about what is best for their patients. Consequently, the clinical trials should provide reliable information concerning endpoints that are relevant to and representative of common practice. The endpoints for evaluating effectiveness should be direct measures of patient welfare, such as survival and symptom control, or cost-effectiveness.

The eligibility criteria used for entry into the study will influence the generalisability of the conclusions. Therefore there are often broad eligibility criteria for phase III clinical trials.

Randomisation

To ensure balance between the arms of the study, patients are randomly allocated to one of the treatment options. This minimises bias and is best conducted by an independent body. There is generally differential bias in the selection of patients to be treated, resulting from judgements by the clinicians, self-selection by the patients and differences in referral patterns. Randomisation does not ensure that the study will include a representative sample of all patients with the disease, but it does help to ensure an unbiased evaluation of the relative merits of the two treatments for the types of patient entered. Randomisation of a patient should be performed after the patient has been found eligible and has consented to participate in the trial and is willing to accept either of the randomised options.

Meta-analysis

A meta-analysis is an exhaustive, objective, quantitative summary of evidence in a particular area. It is focused on quantifying results of individual studies around a focused clinical question, and combines the results from all relevant randomised clinical trials that have been initiated, regardless of whether they have been published. It assesses the therapeutic effectiveness based on the average results pooled across the trials.

A major issue of concern in meta-analyses is whether the individual trials are sufficiently similar to make calculation of average effects that are therapeutically meaningful. A meta-analysis may be useful for answering important questions about a class of treatments that the individual trials cannot address reliably, but it is important to remember that a meta-analysis is not an alternative to properly designed and sized randomised clinical trials.

Table 26.1 Problems encountered in multidisciplinary meetings

Problem	Approach to solution
A team member is absent	Each MDT should appoint a deputy for each core member of the team, such that the meeting functions normally even though a member may be temporarily absent
Addressing patient concerns	It is good practice for the information about the patient's concerns, preferences and social circumstances to be presented at the meeting by someone who has met with the patient, such as a specialist oncology nurse or the treating physician. Where this is at a referring unit, the local staff could join the meeting via teleconference
Decisions not implemented	Studies have shown that 15% of decisions about treatment made at an MDT meeting are not implemented. This frequently results in patients receiving a more conservative treatment than recommended. The main reasons why decisions are not implemented are co-morbid health issues (44%), patient choice (34%) and decisions being changed when more clinical information was available (20%). This reflects the quality and quantity of information available at the time of the meeting, and teams might agree the minimum data required to facilitate discussion of all patients
Inadequate information	MDT meetings require adequate information about the patient's disease as well as any physical or psychological co-morbid health issues
Poor communication	The MDT meeting should record the discussion and recommendations (preferably typed) and communicate the outcome to everyone involved in the management of the patient, including the referring clinician, GP, oncologist, surgeon, radiotherapist, clinical nurse specialist and the patient notes
Poor leadership	MDT meetings can degrade into argumentative confrontations and strong leadership is required. There should be an identified lead person for the meeting and all members should be trained in advanced communication skills and maintain respect for other team members. Regular business meetings should discuss problems and agree approaches to improve the running and efficiency of the meetings

Multidisciplinary team meetings

The multidisciplinary team (MDT) is a group of healthcare professionals who work together to provide high-quality clinical services to patients, increasing efficiency and producing well-rounded care. The core basis of the team is made of up of the health professionals directly involved in the patient's care, such as physicians, specialist nurses and physiotherapists. The wider team encompasses professionals who have an adjunctive role during the patient's journey, such as occupational therapists.

Role of the team

The MDT has become well established in oncology, as cancer is a multisystem disease requiring input from a variety of disciplines. The team meet on a regular basis to discuss the patient's progress and provide a forum for interdisciplinary communication, allowing for coordination of care and decision making. The meeting is designed to be patient centred and provides an opportunity for communication between the different disciplines, planning of investigations and management. It is a platform on which individual clinicians can discuss complex cases or situations and draw on the collective experience of the team membership to decide on the best approach for an individual patient. This can be particularly important when discussing the patients with a rare condition or situation.

Specific roles of the MDT include:
- plan the diagnostic and staging procedures;
- decide on the appropriate primary treatment modality (most commonly surgery but the use of neoadjuvant chemotherapy before interval surgery is increasing);
- arrange review by the oncology team to plan the assessment of the patient prior to systemic therapy or radiotherapy;
- to discuss the additional support requirements for the individual patient, such as physiotherapy, psychological support, symptom control, nutritional care or rehabilitation in the postoperative period;
- ensuring access to accurate information on treatment, prognosis, side effects and other related matters, such as stoma care;
- planning of surveillance strategies;
- ensuring the appropriate transition from treatment with curative intent to that of palliation of symptoms;
- promotion of recruitment into clinical trials;
- agreement of operational policies to deliver high-quality care to patients;
- planning and review of audit data to ensure the delivery of quality care to patients by the team.

Benefit of MDT meetings

Studies have shown that multidisciplinary teams can improve the quality of life, lower mortality and reduce the cost of cancer care. Involvement from an early stage facilitates appropriate and timely treatment, which is more likely to align with evidence-based standards and can lead to greater patient satisfaction. Not only is the multidisciplinary team working well together of great benefit to the patient, it can also benefit the healthcare professionals themselves, with studies showing greater job satisfaction of those involved. The meetings allow interspeciality working, providing a basis for support and education for the whole team. The streamlined care provided by these meetings saves time by improving the coordination between services, reducing duplication of investigations and minimising inefficient communication. On the whole they can make the care more efficient, saving time, money and resources, which inevitably leads to a greater standard of care for the patient and wider benefit to the NHS.

Combined clinics

A number of MDTs run a combined clinic in which several team members are present. Patients can be seen by more than one specialist in the same hospital visit, providing a one-stop opportunity to review and plan treatment. This approach negates the requirement for writing referral letters, improves communication between team members, reduces delays as patients can be reviewed by more than one specialist and is more efficient for the patient. Joint decisions relating to treatment can be decided and implemented in the minimal amount of time, thereby shorting the time to initiation of treatment.

Recruitment into clinical trials

The discussion during MDT meetings to plan the management of patients is an ideal platform to identify potential patients to be considered for clinical trials. The MDT records allow auditing of patient identification, screening and eventual recruitment. In the UK, cancer networks have targets for recruitment into clinical trials. The presence of a research coordinator or research nurse can remind the attendees of the meeting that a particular patient may be eligible for a trial.

The consideration of patients during the MDT meeting has the added benefit of educating all members of the team to the nature, aims and objectives of the study, and clinicians are encouraged to identify scenarios in which there is limited evidence of the optimal management of specific cases to help inform the design and planning of future studies.

Education opportunities

Multidisciplinary teams play a prominent role in the care of patients, therefore students and trainees are encouraged throughout their training to work alongside the MDT and attend meetings.

The educational benefits include:
- examples of interprofessional team working;
- case-based learning, including ethical or psychosocial dilemmas;
- improved knowledge of the disease and management;
- discussion of multimodality management of cancer;
- patient advocacy;
- an opportunity to develop presentation skills;
- discussion of recent research findings and clinical relevance;
- reflections on decision making.

In conclusion, the multidisciplinary meetings can be of very high educational value to all the members involved, especially medical students.

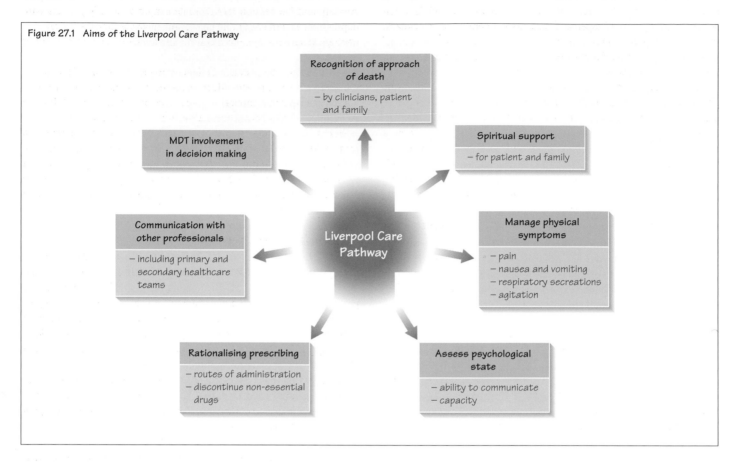

Figure 27.1 Aims of the Liverpool Care Pathway

For patients with incurable malignancies who are reaching the end of life, palliating symptoms and maximising quality of life become the main goals of treatment. Palliative care aims to support those with life-threatening illnesses, including cancers, by addressing all biopsychosocial aspects of their care. This should include support for the patient and their family from the entire multidisciplinary team.

Other chapters have discussed two of the most common problems for palliative patients: nausea and pain. However, there are many other issues that may affect such patients, and controlling them can make a great difference to quality of life.

Physical symptoms

Constipation: there are numerous possible causes for constipation in cancer patients. The most common include drug side effects (particularly with opioid analgesia and anti-emetics), reduced fluid and nutritional intake, intestinal obstruction (due to tumour or strictures) and hypercalcaemia. Mobilisation and increased oral intake can help encourage bowel activity, but often softening or stimulating laxatives need to be administered. When prescribing opioid analgesia, concurrent use of a laxative should always be considered.

Diarrhoea: multiple factors may be involved. Pathogenic causes should be excluded, such as Norovirus or *C. difficile* infection. Drugs that can cause diarrhoea include chemotherapy, NSAIDs, antibiotics and laxatives. Radiotherapy can cause acute and delayed diarrhoea with onset many months after completion of treatment. It is important to identify overflow diarrhoea secondary to constipation, and a rectal examination may be necessary. Removal of the underlying cause is preferable, but if this is not appropriate, treatment with drugs such as loperamide (an opioid receptor agonist) may be beneficial.

Breathlessness: this can be due to many factors, which if reversible should be corrected. Respiratory causes include direct effect of lung tumours, pneumonia, pleural effusion, respiratory muscle weakness, phrenic nerve damage and rib metastases. Cardiovascular causes include congestive cardiac failure, pulmonary embolus, anaemia, arrhythmias and pericardial effusion. Anxiety is an important factor to consider, either as a primary cause or worsening an underlying condition. Oxygen can help if the patient is hypoxic, or even as a placebo to relieve anxiety, and opioids may help to reduce the respiratory rate and calm the patient. Benzodiazepines are useful in reducing anxiety.

Cough: a common symptom in lung cancer due to airway irritation, or as a side effect of drugs including chemotherapy and ACE inhibitors. Treatments include simple linctus which reduces coughing by coating the pharynx, along with opioid-based oral solutions which suppress the cough stimulus.

Cachexia: loss of muscle mass and fat tissue due to increased metabolic demands of an underlying pathology are very common in advanced cancer patients (especially lung and colorectal). Cachexia cannot be reversed by increasing nutritional intake, and is often accompanied by loss of appetite (anorexia) and generalised weakness. It is a poor prognostic indicator that is difficult to influence with treatment. Corticosteroids may stimulate appetite, but cannot prevent further muscle wastage.

Lymphoedema: arises due to damage to or obstruction of the lymphatic system, resulting in chronic oedema often with associated skin changes. Lymphoedema may be inherited (primary) or secondary to damage caused by tumour infiltration, surgery, or radiotherapy. It may affect one or multiple areas, commonly head and neck with mouth or throat cancers, upper limbs with breast cancer and lower limbs with colorectal or gynaecological cancers. Preventive treatment is preferable, in addition to referral to a specialist lymphoedema service. Treatments includes tissue massage, compression bandages or garments and skin care. Cellulitis is a common complication in cancer patients, and patient education on warning signs is essential.

Mouthcare: the mouth is particularly at risk of complications in cancer patients. Dry mouth is very common and often due to anticholinergic drugs, chemotherapy or radiotherapy, in addition to dehydration. Chemotherapy or radiotherapy may cause mucositis, painful mucosal inflammation which makes the mouth vulnerable to infection. Candidiasis is common and can be treated with local sprays (e.g. nystatin) or systemic agents (e.g. fluconazole). Good oral hygiene is essential to prevent bacterial, viral and fungal infection, and antibiotic or chlorhexidine mouthwash may be used alongside normal tooth cleaning. Artificial saliva is beneficial to some patients.

Psychological issues

Distress: most patients with a terminal diagnosis undergo some degree of emotional distress. Multiple factors may be responsible for this distress and it is important to attempt to address as many as possible. Good communication skills are vital when discussing prognosis with the patient and family, incorporating both honesty and reassurance where appropriate. Involving the patient and family in decisions about their care and respecting patient autonomy is essential. Control of physical symptoms can be of great benefit to a patient's mental state.

Depression: is common in end of life patients and it is crucial to distinguish normal psychological distress from significant clinical depression. Physical symptoms of depression such as lack of energy and loss of appetite may be masked by the biological progression of cancer. However, appropriate screening tools such as the Hospital Anxiety and Depression (HAD) scale can help identify patients with depression. Treatment should be holistic, incorporating additional psychological support, symptom control and antidepressant medication if necessary.

Spirituality: the patient's beliefs, thoughts, hopes and fears about the end of their life should be explored with them to ensure that appropriate spiritual support is given. This includes, but is not limited to, religious faiths and cultural ideas around death and dying.

Bereavement: support for patients and their families coming to terms with the prospect of dying is important. Grief can develop both before and after a death, and informal support, as well as psychological therapy, can be very beneficial. Cancer support groups are extremely helpful in helping patients and relatives understand the disease and deal with its consequences.

Managing the terminal phase

In the final days and hours of life, frameworks such as the Liverpool Care Pathway (LCP) can aid clinicians in ensuring completeness and consistency of care (Figure 27.1). Active treatment is usually no longer part of medical care in the terminal phase. The place of care is important, as dying patients may be cared for at home, in nursing care, in hospital, or in a hospice. Statistically, most cancer patients will die in hospital, but the patient's choice of location should be facilitated if at all possible, providing medical needs can be met.

Prescribing in the most terminal stages should include essential medications only, and routes of administration that minimise discomfort should be prioritised. For example, choosing to give pain relief via subcutaneous syringe drivers rather than intravenously or orally.

Withdrawal of nutrition and hydration may be appropriate once it is clear that the patient is in the final hours of life. This can be distressing for family members, but should not be uncomfortable for the patient. This should be discussed carefully and explained with both the patient and family. Intravenous fluid and non-oral nutrition are invasive treatments, often with little benefit in the terminal phase. Fluid withdrawal may improve respiratory secretions, pulmonary oedema and cerebral oedema, and make the patient's dying process more comfortable.

28 Carcinoma of unknown primary

Figure 28.1 Clinical features of unknown primary cancer

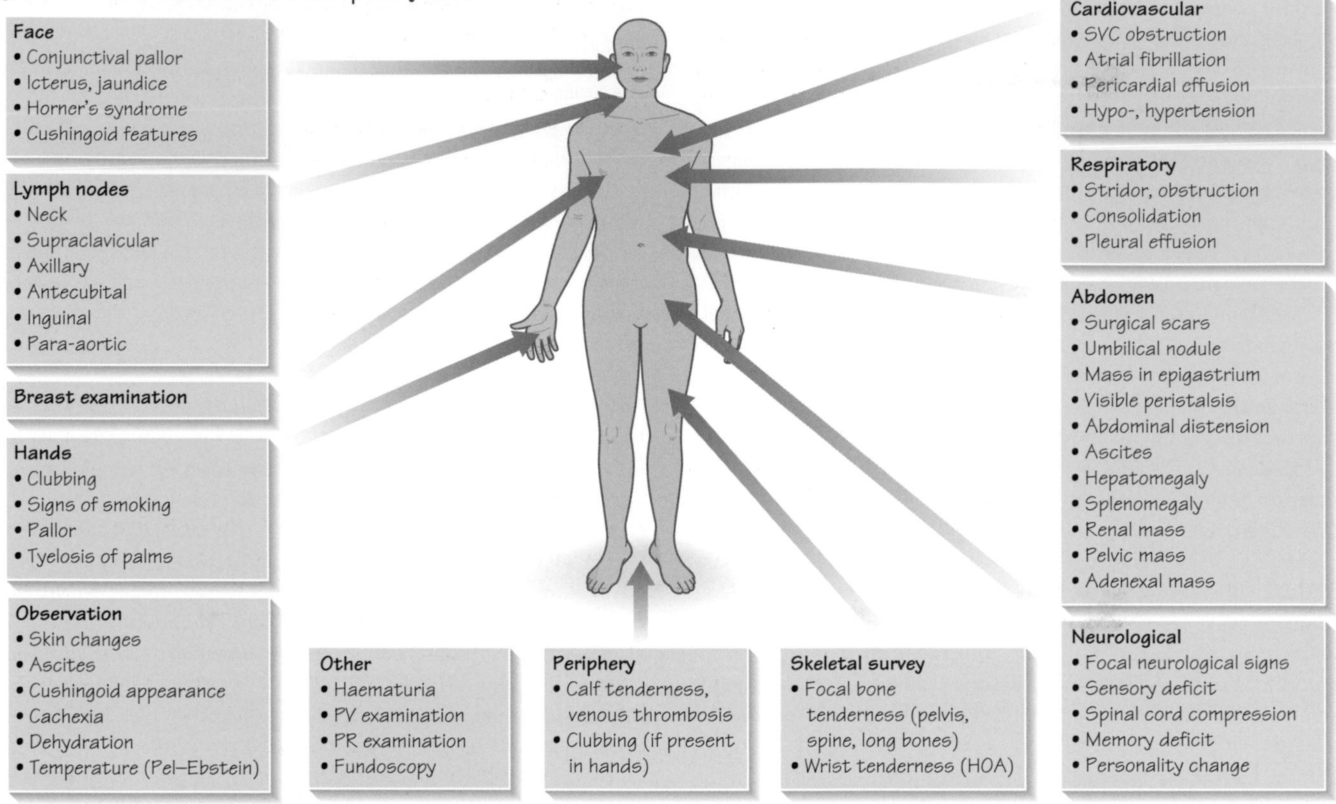

Face
- Conjunctival pallor
- Icterus, jaundice
- Horner's syndrome
- Cushingoid features

Lymph nodes
- Neck
- Supraclavicular
- Axillary
- Antecubital
- Inguinal
- Para-aortic

Breast examination

Hands
- Clubbing
- Signs of smoking
- Pallor
- Tyelosis of palms

Observation
- Skin changes
- Ascites
- Cushingoid appearance
- Cachexia
- Dehydration
- Temperature (Pel–Ebstein)

Other
- Haematuria
- PV examination
- PR examination
- Fundoscopy

Periphery
- Calf tenderness, venous thrombosis
- Clubbing (if present in hands)

Skeletal survey
- Focal bone tenderness (pelvis, spine, long bones)
- Wrist tenderness (HOA)

Cardiovascular
- SVC obstruction
- Atrial fibrillation
- Pericardial effusion
- Hypo-, hypertension

Respiratory
- Stridor, obstruction
- Consolidation
- Pleural effusion

Abdomen
- Surgical scars
- Umbilical nodule
- Mass in epigastrium
- Visible peristalsis
- Abdominal distension
- Ascites
- Hepatomegaly
- Splenomegaly
- Renal mass
- Pelvic mass
- Adenexal mass

Neurological
- Focal neurological signs
- Sensory deficit
- Spinal cord compression
- Memory deficit
- Personality change

Table 28.1 Common sites of involvement

Site	Incidence as first site of metastasis (%)	Incidence of involvement at presentation (%)
Lymph node	26	41
Lung	17	27
Bone	15	29
Liver	11	34
Brain	8	6
Pleura	7	11
Skin	5	4
Peritoneum	4	9
Adrenal gland	–	6
Bone marrow	–	3

Table 28.2
Approach to patients

Step 1	Search for a primary site
Step 2	Rule out potentially treatable or curable tumours
Step 3	Characterise the specific clinicopathological entity and then treat the patient • favourable subsets should consider curative intent • unfavourable subsets require palliative intent

Table 28.4
Malignancies that can be identified by immunohistochemistry

- Neuroendocrine tumours
- Lymphomas
- Germ cell tumours
- Melanomas
- Sarcomas
- Serous tumours (ovarian, peritoneal, uterine)
- Embryonal malignancies (especially in childhood)

Table 28.3 Light microscopy can classify CUP

- Well to moderately differentiated adenocarcinoma (50%)
- Poorly or undifferentiated adenocarcinoma (30%)
- Squamous cell carcinoma (15%)
- Undifferentiated carcinoma (5%)

Epidemiology

Cancer will often present as a result of symptoms due to the primary site of the tumour, but sometimes the cancer is able to metastasise before the primary site is large enough to be detected. In contrast to known primary tumours, carcinomas of unknown primary (CUP) tend to have early dissemination, unpredictable metastatic pattern, aggressive nature and an absence of symptoms from the primary site. CUP is therefore defined as the detection of one or more sites of metastatic tumours for which investigations have failed to identify the primary site.

Up to 5% of all cancers are from an unknown primary, representing eight to 20 patients per 100 000 of the population per year. It is the seventh most frequent form of cancer and fourth most common cause of cancer death in both males and females. The median age at presentation is 60 years and 50% of patients present with multiple sites of involvement, with the rest having a single site in: liver, bones, lungs, or lymph nodes.

Aetiology

The usual histological diagnosis is that of adenocarcinoma or poorly differentiated carcinoma. Different tumours will spread in different patterns and this may be related to the chemokine and chemokine receptor expression by the tumour and stromal cells.

Clinical presentation

The clinical presentation will depend on the location of disease sites, but most patients (97%) have symptoms at metastatic sites (Table 28.1). Non-specific symptoms such as anorexia, weight loss and fatigue are common. See Chapter 10 for approach to clinical examination.

Investigations and staging

The first consideration is to exclude a potentially curable tumour, then to identify tumour types that are associated with a more favourable outcome, due to their responsiveness to treatment (Table 28.2). Despite extensive investigation, fewer than 20% of patients have a primary site identified antemortem, and even at autopsy 70% of cases have an unidentified primary site.

Primary sites are most frequently detected in the lung and pancreas, followed by other gastrointestinal and gynaecological malignancies.

Initial investigations

- Complete history and physical examination
- Full blood count
- Serum biochemistry and liver function
- Serum tumour markers (see Chapter 15)
- Urinalysis, stool testing for occult blood
- Chest X-ray
- Symptom-directed endoscopy
- Imaging of thorax, abdomen and pelvis (CT, MRI, or PET)
- Plain film imaging of bone pain sites
- Biopsy for histology (any site of disease) (Tables 28.3 and 28.4)

Patients should be referred to an oncologist who can advise on the required investigations, as there should be concern about overinvestigating the patient. This will have a cost effect and potentially can delay the initiation of appropriate treatment for the patient. Therefore a limited diagnostic approach with patient-benefit orientation aiming to recognise patients with good prognostic features is the best approach.

It is possible for patients to deteriorate during the investigation period and a precise diagnosis of the primary site may not be possible. Therefore, an approach is required that balances the need for sufficient tests to plan the management versus treatment of the disease.

Treatment

For patients with an incurable malignancy that is widely metastatic, treatment with combination systemic chemotherapy is the most appropriate. The choice of treatment will depend on the best assessment of likely primary site and consideration of the performance status of the patient. Radiotherapy is useful for specific sites of pain or discomfort. All treatment is administered with palliative intent and the aim of improving the patient's quality of life. Furthermore, treatments should be discontinued if the patient is no longer gaining benefit or improvement in symptoms.

For patients with well or moderated differentiated adenocarcinoma of unknown primary, 90% demonstrate a low response rate to chemotherapy. Patients in this group have a poor prognosis.

Patients with potential ovarian or peritoneal primary sites can respond very well with appropriate chemotherapy; 40% achieve complete remission and 20% can achieve prolonged disease-free survival. Patients with axillary lymph node metastasis can be treated as for breast cancer and may require modified radical mastectomy.

Patients with poorly differentiated carcinoma or adenocarcinoma account for 30% of patients with CUP. They demonstrate a poor response to systemic chemotherapy, have a poor outcome and short survival. Such patients have a younger median age (40 years) and a rapid progression of symptoms. The most common sites of involvement include lymph nodes, mediastinum and retroperitoneum. Rarely, excellent responses and improved survival are demonstrated but no identified factors can predict response in these patients.

For patients with a single site of metastasis, consideration should be made for surgical resection and treatment with radiotherapy. This can produce significant periods of disease-free survival in some patients.

The presence of osteoblastic bone metastasis in a male patient should be considered for empirical hormonal therapy as for prostate cancer, regardless of the serum PSA level.

Prognosis

Patients with a diagnosis of carcinoma of unknown primary have a limited life expectancy with a median survival of 6–9 months. Patients with one to two sites of involvement, non-adenocarcinoma and no involvement of liver, bone, or adrenal gland have a median survival of 40 months. For patients with adrenal metastasis it is 5 months. Adverse prognostic factors include:

- adenocarcinoma histology;
- increasing number of involved organ sites;
- hepatic or adrenal involvement;
- supraclavicular lymph node involvement;
- male gender;
- poor performance status;
- weight loss (>10% of body mass).

29 Breast cancer

Figure 29.1 Clinical features of breast cancer

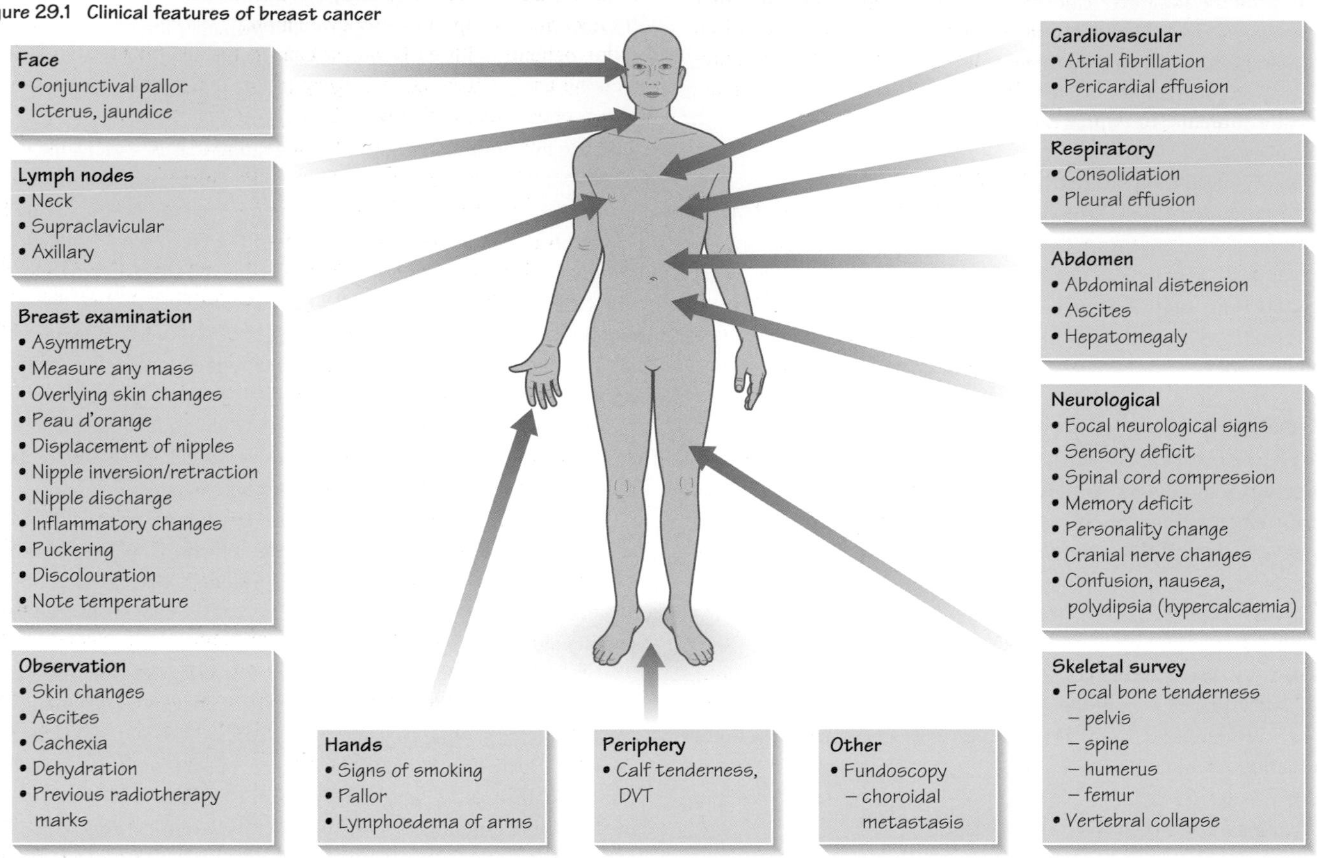

Face
- Conjunctival pallor
- Icterus, jaundice

Lymph nodes
- Neck
- Supraclavicular
- Axillary

Breast examination
- Asymmetry
- Measure any mass
- Overlying skin changes
- Peau d'orange
- Displacement of nipples
- Nipple inversion/retraction
- Nipple discharge
- Inflammatory changes
- Puckering
- Discolouration
- Note temperature

Observation
- Skin changes
- Ascites
- Cachexia
- Dehydration
- Previous radiotherapy marks

Hands
- Signs of smoking
- Pallor
- Lymphoedema of arms

Periphery
- Calf tenderness, DVT

Other
- Fundoscopy
  - choroidal metastasis

Cardiovascular
- Atrial fibrillation
- Pericardial effusion

Respiratory
- Consolidation
- Pleural effusion

Abdomen
- Abdominal distension
- Ascites
- Hepatomegaly

Neurological
- Focal neurological signs
- Sensory deficit
- Spinal cord compression
- Memory deficit
- Personality change
- Cranial nerve changes
- Confusion, nausea, polydipsia (hypercalcaemia)

Skeletal survey
- Focal bone tenderness
  - pelvis
  - spine
  - humerus
  - femur
- Vertebral collapse

Table 29.1 TNM staging of breast cancer

Classification	Division	Description
T – extent of tumour	T0	No evidence of primary tumour
	T1	Tumour 2cm or less in its greatest dimension **a.** no fixation to underlying pectoral muscle or fascia **b.** fixation to underlying muscle or fascia
	T2	Tumour more than 2cm but not more than 5cm in its greatest dimension
	T3	Tumour more than 5cm in its greatest dimension **a.** no fixation to underlying pectoral muscle or fascia **b.** fixation to underlying muscle or fascia
	T4	Tumour of any size fixed with direct extension to chest wall or skin Note: chest wall includes ribs, intercostal muscles and serratus anterior muscle, but not pectoral muscle
N – regional lymph nodes	N0	No ipsilateral lymph node metastasis
	N1	Movable ipsilateral axillary nodes **a.** nodes not considered to contain growth **b.** nodes considered to contain growth
	N2	Ipsilateral axillary nodes containing growth and fixed to one another or to other structures
	N3	Ipsilateral supraclavicular or infraclavicular nodes containing growth or oedema of the arm
M – metastasis	M0	No distant metastasis
	M1	Distant metastasis present, including skin involvement beyond the breast area

Epidemiology

Breast cancer is the most frequent cancer in women after non-melanotic skin tumours (32% of female cancers) and is the commonest cause of death in women aged 35–54 years in England. It follows an unpredictable course with metastases presenting up to 20 years after initial diagnosis. England has one of the highest age-standardised incidences and mortality from breast cancer in the world, with a life-time risk of breast cancer of 1 in 9. Earlier detection by screening and improved treatment are improving the 5-year survival.

Aetiology and pathophysiology

Both genetic and hormonal factors play a role in the aetiology of breast cancer. Hereditary predisposition is implicated in around 10% of breast cancer cases, including *BRCA1* and *BRCA2* hereditary breast cancer, and Li–Fraumeni syndrome. Prolonged exposure to oestrogen is thought to play a role and early menarche, late menopause, late first pregnancy (over 35 years old) and nulliparity are established risk factors.

The combined oral contraceptive pill does not significantly increase the relative risk for breast cancer (see Chapter 3), but hormone replacement therapy (HRT) has been shown to increase the incidence of breast cancer in long-term current users (relative risk 1.66).

Invasive ductal carcinoma with or without ductal carcinoma in situ (DCIS) is the commonest histology, accounting for 70% of cases, while invasive lobular carcinoma accounts for most of the remaining cases. DCIS constitutes 20% of screening-detected breast cancers, is multifocal in one-third of women and has a high risk of becoming invasive (10% at 5 years following excision only). Pure DCIS does not cause lymph node metastases, although these are found in 2% of cases where nodes are examined, owing to undetected invasive cancer. Lobular carcinoma in situ (LCIS) is a predisposing risk factor for developing cancer in either breast (7% at 10 years).

Clinical presentation

Breast cancer usually presents as a mass that persists throughout the menstrual cycle. A nipple discharge occurs in 10% and pain in only 7% of patients. Less common presentations include inflammatory carcinoma with diffuse induration of the skin of the breast, and this confers an adverse prognosis. Increasingly, women present as a consequence of mammographic screening. About 40% of patients will have axillary nodal disease, the likelihood of this rising with increasing size of the primary tumour. The involvement of axillary nodes by tumour is the strongest prognostic predictor. Distant metastases are infrequently present at diagnosis and the commonest sites of spread are: bone (70%), lung (60%), liver (55%), pleura (40%), adrenals (35%), skin (30%) and brain (10–20%).

Paget's disease of the nipple accounts for 1% of all breast cancer cases and presents with a relatively long history of eczematous change in the nipple area with itching, burning, oozing, or bleeding. There may be a palpable underlying lump. The nipple contains malignant cells singularly or in nests. Prognosis is related to the underlying tumour.

Treatment

The management of **carcinoma in situ** is not well defined, as surgery with simple mastectomy or breast-conserving surgery followed by radiotherapy yield higher relapse rates, but salvage mastectomy at relapse can produce similar survival rates. The suggested treatment options for LCIS span from observation with annual screening to bilateral prophylactic mastectomy in selected patients. There appears to be no place for chemotherapy in either DCIS or LCIS, and the role of endocrine therapy is under evaluation.

For patients with early breast cancer, the treatment is wide local excision and axillary node surgery (dissection, sampling, or sentinel lymph node biopsy) followed by adjuvant breast radiotherapy. This achieves similar local control and survival rates to mastectomy with less mutilating surgery. **Adjuvant radiotherapy** is given to reduce the risk of local recurrence. This is reduced from 40–60% to 4–6% with the use of postoperative radiotherapy.

Adjuvant hormonal therapy with tamoxifen and aromatase inhibitors can improve disease-free and overall survival in pre- and post-menopausal patients who have tumours that express the oestrogen receptor (ER+). Patients at low risk with tumours that are small and ER+ require only adjuvant hormonal therapy. Patients with tumours that are ER+ and who are pre-menopausal should receive a luteinising hormone releasing hormone (LHRH) analogue, and postmenopausal patients, tamoxifen and an aromatase inhibitor.

Adjuvant chemotherapy is considered for patients at higher risk of recurrence. Factors that increase the risk of recurrence include a tumour >1 cm, tumour that is oestrogen receptor negative (ER–) or the presence of involved axillary lymph nodes. Such patients should be offered adjuvant chemotherapy, which improves disease-free and overall survival. The role of adjuvant treatment has been studied by meta-analyses and data supports the use of adjuvant trastuzumab, a humanised monoclonal antibody to HER2, in addition to standard chemotherapy for women with early HER2+ breast cancer.

The aim is to personalise the treatment approach for ER+, ER/PR/HER 'triple' negative patients and those who are HER2+. The clinico-pathological behaviour of these groups of patients is distinct and they require appropriate treatment strategies to optimise the survival benefits of adjuvant treatment.

Metastatic disease management includes radiotherapy to palliate painful bone metastases, and second-line endocrine therapy with aromatase inhibitors, which inhibit peripheral oestrogen production in adrenal and adipose tissues. Advanced ER– disease may be treated with combination chemotherapy and trastuzumab may be considered for patients with relapsed HER2+ disease. Bisphosphonates can treat hypercalcaemia and reduce skeletal morbidity in women with bone metastases.

Prevention

Chemoprevention with tamoxifen has been shown to reduce the incidence of breast cancer in an American randomised controlled trial of 13 000 healthy women at high risk of developing breast cancer. However, these results have not been reproduced in two similar European trials.

Screening

Breast cancer screening is discussed in Chapter 16.

Figure 30.1 Clinical features of lung cancer

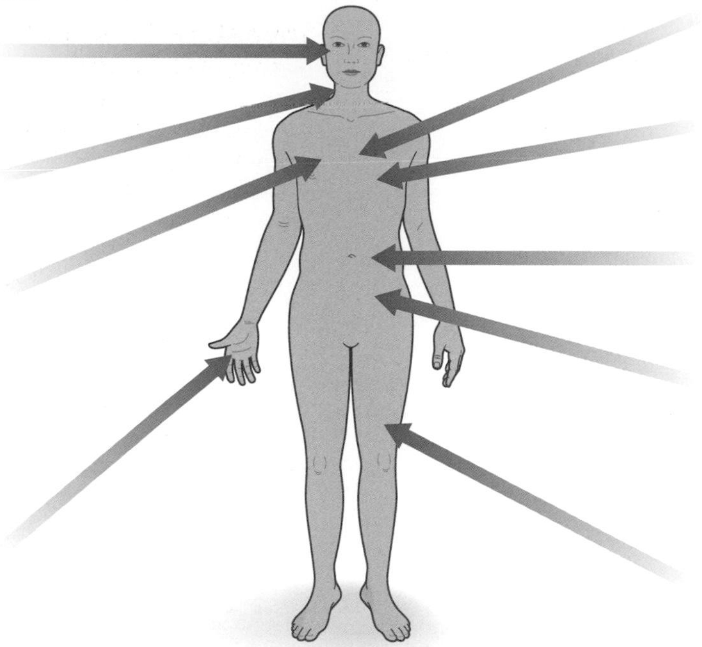

Face
- Conjunctival pallor
- Icterus, jaundice
- Horner's syndrome
- Cushingoid features

Lymph nodes
- Neck
- Supraclavicular
- Axillary

Symptoms
- Persistent cough
- Haemoptysis
- Chest pain
- Hoarseness of voice (recurrent laryngeal nerve)
- Breathlessness
- Dysphagia
- Shoulder pain (brachial plexus involvement)

Hands
- Clubbing
- Signs of smoking
- Pallor
- Wasting of small muscles (T1 root compression)

Periphery
- Clubbing (if present in hands)
- Ankle tenderness (HOA)

Observation
- Ascites
- Cushingoid appearance
- Cachexia
- Dehydration
- Fatigue
- Anorexia
- Gynaecomastia

Cardiovascular
- SVC obstruction
- Atrial fibrillation
- Pericardial effusion

Respiratory
- Tachypnoea
- Stridor
- Consolidation
- Pleural effusion

Abdomen
- Abdominal distension
- Ascites
- Hepatomegaly

Neurological
- Confusion
- Focal neurological signs
- Sensory deficit
- Spinal cord compression
- Memory deficit
- Personality change
- Hallucinations

Skeletal survey
- Focal bone tenderness
- Pathological fracture (pelvis, spine, long bones)
- Wrist tenderness (HOA)

Other
- Weight loss
- Spirometry

Table 30.1 TNM staging of non-small cell lung cancer

Classification	Division	Description
T – extent of tumour	Tx	Primary tumour that cannot be assessed, may be confirmed by malignant cells in sputum or bronchial washings but not visualised on imaging
	Tis	No evidence of primary tumour
	T0	Carcinoma in situ
	T1	Tumour <3 cm surrounded by lung or visceral pleura, without evidence of more proximal invasion than the lobar bronchus
	T2	Tumour >3 cm, or in main bronchus, >2 cm distal to carina or invading visceral pleura or associated with atelectasis or obstructive pneumonitis that extends to the hilar region, but does not involve whole lung
	T3	Tumour of any size that invades chest wall, diaphragm, parietal pericardium, mediastinal pleura, or tumour in main bronchus <2 cm distal to carina, or associated atelectasis or obstructive pneumonitis of the entire lung
	T4	Tumour of any size invading mediastinum, heart, great vessels, trachea, oesophagus, carina, vertebral body, or separate nodules in the ipsilateral lobe
N – regional lymph nodes	Nx	Cannot be assessed
	N0	No regional lymph node metastasis
	N1	Ipsilateral peribronchial and/or ipsilateral hilar nodes and intrapulmonary nodes involved by direct extension of tumour
	N2	Ipsilateral mediastinal and/or subcarinal nodes
	N3	Contralateral mediastinal, hilar nodes, or any scalene or supraclavicular nodes
M – metastasis	Mx	Cannot be assessed
	M0	No distant metastasis
	M1	Distant metastasis present, including separate nodules in different lobes

Epidemiology

Lung cancer is the most common cancer worldwide and the second most common in the UK, with 41 000 new cases per year (13% of all new cancer diagnosis). The majority (87%) are in people over 65 years, with the highest incidence between 80 and 84 years and the lowest in people under 40. There has been a demographic shift, with the incidence and mortality rates falling in males and rising in females. Despite government initiatives to reduce smoking rates, lung cancer remains the biggest cause of cancer deaths in the UK and USA.

Aetiology

The most significant risk factor for lung cancer is smoking (80–90% of cases, RR = 17), including passive smoking (RR = 1.5). The risk is proportional to the patient's pack years (packs smoked per day × years smoked), the age they started and the type of cigarette smoked. Other recognised risk factors include previous radiotherapy to the chest, and occupational exposure to chemicals such as asbestos, acetaldehyde, beryllium, cadmium, chromium, formaldehyde, polycyclic aromatic hydrocarbons, nickel and inorganic arsenic compounds.

There is a 2.5-fold increased risk of lung cancer where there is a significant family history, despite their own smoking history, and rarely lung cancers develop in patients with germ line mutations in genes such as in *Rb* and *TP53*.

Pathophysiology

Small cell lung cancer (SCLC) accounts for 20% of all lung cancers and arises in the larger airways; it tends to be a more central tumour. Most patients present with systemic disease and it frequently metastasises, via haematogenous spread, to the liver, skeleton, bone marrow, brain and adrenal glands. The small cells contain dense neurosecretory granules which can produce ectopic biological substances resulting in Cushing's syndrome (ACTH) and SIAD. Mutations in *RB1* and *TP53* are found in 80% of patients with SCLC and abnormal DNA methylation of the cyclin D2 gene is common.

Non-small cell lung cancers (NSCLC) (80% of lung cancers) arise from the epithelial cells of the lung from the central bronchi to the terminal alveoli. They can be divided into three main types.
- **Squamous cell carcinoma** (50%) is the commonest histological diagnosis, often presenting as an obstructive lesion of the bronchus, causing infection. They can cavitate on a chest radiograph and tend to grow slowly, spreading locally and disseminating late.
- **Adenocarcinoma** (15%) arises from the bronchial mucosal glands and tends to occur in the periphery. As such findings can represent a metastasis from a distant site, careful patient assessment is required. There is less association with smoking, but they can originate in scar tissue and carry a high risk of metastatic spread, often to mediastinal lymph nodes and pleura producing an effusion.
- **Large cell carcinoma** (10%) often presents as a large peripheral mass on a chest radiograph and can have neurosecretory elements that produce paraneoplastic features. They tend to be poorly differentiated, can grow rapidly and metastasise early.

Clinical presentation

Patients can present asymptomatic but the majority present with a cough (41%). Other common symptoms include chest pain, haemoptysis, breathlessness and recurrent chest infections. Finger clubbing is particularly common in NSCLC.

Local spread can result in lymphadenopathy, dysphagia, hoarseness of the voice (recurrent laryngeal nerve involvement) and shoulder pain. Metastases can present with bone pain, liver discomfort and neurological signs due to CNS involvement. Extrathoracic symptoms include anorexia, weight loss, malaise and lethargy.

Paraneoplastic syndromes are particularly associated with lung cancer, including dermatomyositis, acanthosis nigricans, LEMS and ectopic production of ACTH, ADH and PTHrP (see Chapter 11).

Investigations and staging

The aim of investigation is to gain a histological diagnosis and determine the extent of spread (stage), and should include a chest X-ray, full blood count, liver function tests and serum calcium. Sputum cytology can be unreliable. CT imaging is used to assess the tumour size and spread, determine lymph node involvement or identify chest wall invasion or metastasis to other sites.

Tissue for diagnostic testing is usually obtained during a bronchoscopy, but an FNA of involved lymph nodes or CT-guided biopsy may be considered. Fluid cytology from a pleural effusion can be useful. If bone pain is present plain X-rays and bone scan imaging are required to exclude metastasis.

PET/CT is increasingly being used as an alternative to an invasive mediastinoscopy to determine operability of the patient.

Treatment

In **SCLC**, surgery has a limited role and chemotherapy is required, using etoposide combined with carboplatin or cisplatin, delivered at 3-weekly intervals for four to six cycles. Although there is a high response rate (80–90%, limited stage, 60–80%, extensive stage), most patients relapse and median survival improvement is only 14 months. Radiotherapy can be used as a concurrent therapy with curative intent; for palliation, as 60% of relapses occur within the thorax; or as prophylactic cranial irradiation for patients treated with curative intent, to reduce the risk of CNS metastasis.

NSCLC treatment is dependent on the patient and the type and stage of the cancer. For stages 1, 2 and some 3a patients, complete surgical excision offers the best curative option, often followed by adjuvant chemotherapy. The aim of surgery is to remove the primary tumour with all locoregional lymph nodes, but patients require sufficient fitness and respiratory function to be able to undergo this.

Patients with stage 3b or 4 disease are inoperable and chemotherapy can provide improvement in symptoms and control of disease. Treatment is for four to six cycles using a doublet of carboplatin or cisplatin with gemcitabine or vinorelbine. Forty per cent of patients respond but there are limited survival gains of 6–7 weeks. Second-line therapy is with docetaxel. EGFR tyrosine kinase inhibitors (gefitinib, erlotinib) can be offered to patients with EGFR mutations.

Radiotherapy can be used in a radical or palliative setting. High-dose curative therapy can be given using a schedule of continuous hyperfractionated accelerated radiotherapy (CHART), delivered in three fractions per day for 12 days. High-dose palliative radiotherapy is given over 6 weeks to patients with symptomatic disease, no metastatic spread and a good performance status. Palliative radiotherapy can be useful for symptom control, in particular to improve pain, haemoptysis, breathlessness and cough.

Patients with SVC obstruction should be considered for stent insertion or radiotherapy. Fifty per cent of patients with SVC obstruction will have SCLC, and prompt responses to chemotherapy are common.

For patients with paraneoplastic syndromes due to ectopic production of hormones (e.g. SIAD), the syndrome features will improve if the treatment for the underlying cancer is successful. A return of symptoms of ectopic hormone production should be considered as possible relapse and investigated accordingly.

31 Mesothelioma

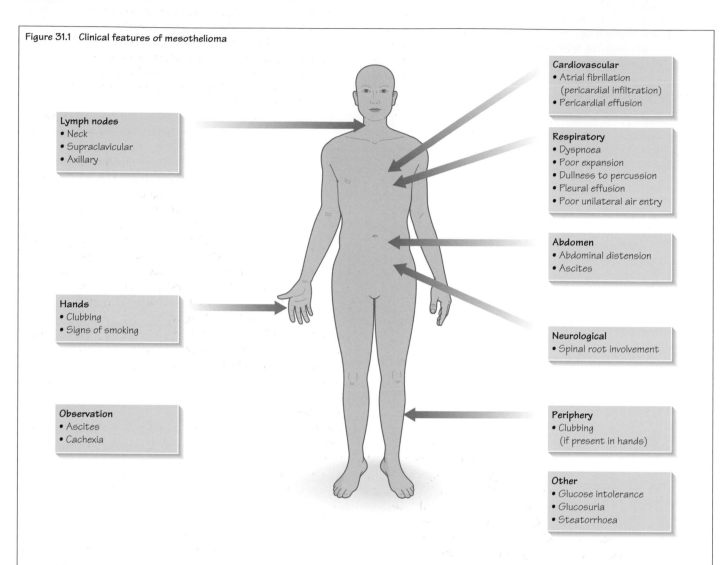

Figure 31.1 Clinical features of mesothelioma

Lymph nodes
• Neck
• Supraclavicular
• Axillary

Hands
• Clubbing
• Signs of smoking

Observation
• Ascites
• Cachexia

Cardiovascular
• Atrial fibrillation (pericardial infiltration)
• Pericardial effusion

Respiratory
• Dyspnoea
• Poor expansion
• Dullness to percussion
• Pleural effusion
• Poor unilateral air entry

Abdomen
• Abdominal distension
• Ascites

Neurological
• Spinal root involvement

Periphery
• Clubbing (if present in hands)

Other
• Glucose intolerance
• Glucosuria
• Steatorrhoea

Table 31.1 Staging of mesothelioma

Stage	Tumour location
I	Tumour involving the right or left pleura and may have spread to the lung, pericardium, or diaphragm on the same side. Lymph nodes are not involved
II	Tumour has spread from the pleura on one side to nearby lymph nodes next to the lung on the same side. It may have spread into the lung, pericardium, or diaphragm on the same side
III	Tumour is invading the chest wall, muscle, ribs, heart, oesophagus, or other organs in the chest on the same side with or without spread to lymph nodes on the same side as the primary tumour
IV	Tumour involving lymph nodes in the chest on the side opposite the primary tumour, or extends to the pleura or lung on the opposite side, or directly extends into organs in the abdominal cavity or neck. Any distant metastases are included in this stage

Epidemiology

Mesothelioma presents at a median age of 60 years, typically 20–50 years after asbestos exposure and affects men five times more than women. Risk has been estimated to be linearly proportional to the intensity and duration of exposure. Latency periods between first exposure to asbestos and a diagnosis of mesothelioma may therefore vary by occupation, with shorter intervals for insulators and dock workers and longer intervals for shipyard and maritime workers, as well as domestic exposures.

A significant proportion of patients with mesothelioma diagnosed between the ages of 20 and 40 report household or neighbourhood exposure during childhood. Children who present with the disease generally have no apparent asbestos exposure. Despite increasing awareness of the role of asbestos in these tumours and measures to reduce asbestos exposure, it is estimated the incidence of mesothelioma will continue to rise until 2020.

Aetiology

Malignant mesothelioma is a rare tumour (<1% of cancers) that is highly aggressive, arising primarily from the surface serosal cells of the pleural, peritoneal and pericardial cavities. Exposure to asbestos fibres is the primary cause, although 50% of patients have no history of exposure. The risk is greatest with blue asbestos (crocidolite) then brown asbestos (amosite) and least with white asbestos (chrysolite).

In 60–83% of human malignant mesotheliomas the cells contain and express SV40 DNA, suggesting a possible co-factor. The exposure to asbestos fibres can produce reactive oxygen species when hydrogen peroxide and superoxide react to form hydroxyl radicals, which can induce DNA damage.

Clinical presentation

More than 90% of patients present with intrathoracic symptoms, such as cough, dyspnoea and non-pleuritic chest wall pain. Involvement of the mediastinal pleural can produce arrhythmias or dysphagia, but these are rare. Pyrexia of unknown origin, sweats, anorexia and weight loss are frequent; thrombocytosis, disseminated intravascular coagulation, thrombophlebitis and haemolytic anaemia can occur.

Most patients present with dullness at one lung base and a unilateral pleural effusion seen on a chest X-ray. Occasional patients are asymptomatic with an effusion simply as an incidental finding. Fewer than 5% have bilateral involvement at the time of diagnosis and 60% have right-sided lesions. The tumour often encases and compresses the lung and spread is predominantly by local invasion of the lung extending into the fissures and interlobular septa, adjacent organs in the mediastinum and chest wall, and may track along chest drainage sites. Thoracic lymph nodes invasion is seen in up to 70% of patients and haematogenous metastases are documented to liver and lung, and less commonly to kidney, adrenal and, rarely, bone.

Investigations and staging

On a chest X-ray mesothelioma appears as a thickened, nodular, irregular pleural-based mass, which covers the pleural surface, and in some patients pleural plaques are visible due to previous asbestos exposure. The tumour often encompasses the involved lung, but is rarely seen bilaterally. Chest wall, diaphragmatic and mediastinal invasion may be seen in advanced cases. Moderate to large pleural effusion is often noted on the affected side.

Using CT imaging, the extent of disease can be assessed (Table 31.1). Pleural thickening >1 cm is seen in most cases (92%), thickening which extends into the interlobular fissure is seen in 85% of cases, pleural effusions in 74% and pleural calcifications in 20–50%. Absence of pleural thickening does not exclude mesothelioma, and the only finding might be pleural effusion. CT imaging can differentiate benign from malignant pleural thickening, but does not reliably distinguish primary from metastatic malignancy.

Pulmonary function tests may show a restrictive lung pattern resulting from encasement of the lung. Obstructive spirometric changes are unrelated to mesothelioma or asbestosis.

Cytology assessment of the pleural fluid is of limited value in mesothelioma, as many will have false negative results (80%). Even with a positive result, many patients still require a biopsy.

A percutaneous needle biopsy of the pleura or peritoneum can be performed under local anaesthetic to obtain a tissue sample, but is diagnostic in only 60% of patients with mesothelioma. The remainder require an open biopsy, which is more reliable and provides a larger tissue specimen for assessment. Increasingly, a video-assisted thoracoscopic (VAT) approach is used and as recurrent pleural effusions are common, a talc pleurodesis with pleural stripping can be performed at the same time as the VAT biopsy.

Tumour seeding may occur along the needle tract of a biopsy and in approximately 20% of patients tumour nodules develop at the biopsy site. Local radiotherapy to the biopsy site may prevent nodule growth.

Treatment

Unfortunately, the majority of patients with mesothelioma present with incurable disease. Analgesics for chest pain, antibiotics for infection and cough suppressants can all palliate symptoms and should be considered. The approach to surgery and systemic treatments is usually palliative, as cure is unlikely unless patients present with localised disease that is resected.

Occasionally patients have operable stage 1 disease with tumour confined to the ipsilateral pleural space, when either decortication (pleurectomy) or extrapleural pneumonectomy may be performed followed by adjuvant radiotherapy. The extent of benefit from surgery has not been established through randomised clinical trials. Radiotherapy may be used for more advanced disease to control symptoms, and palliation can be achieved with systemic chemotherapy using carboplatin (or cisplatin) and pemetrexed. Radiotherapy is used to control metastasis at port sites following invasive procedures and to prevent growth at such sites.

Drainage of pleural or pericardial effusion and pleurodesis may control symptoms due to effusion.

Prognosis

The 5-year survival for mesothelioma is 5%, with survival ranging from 6 to 18 months. In the UK, patients with asbestos-related mesothelioma are eligible for a lump sum payment in addition to their other benefit entitlements and they should be directed to appropriate advice.

32 Oesophageal cancer

Figure 32.1 Clinical features of oesophageal cancer

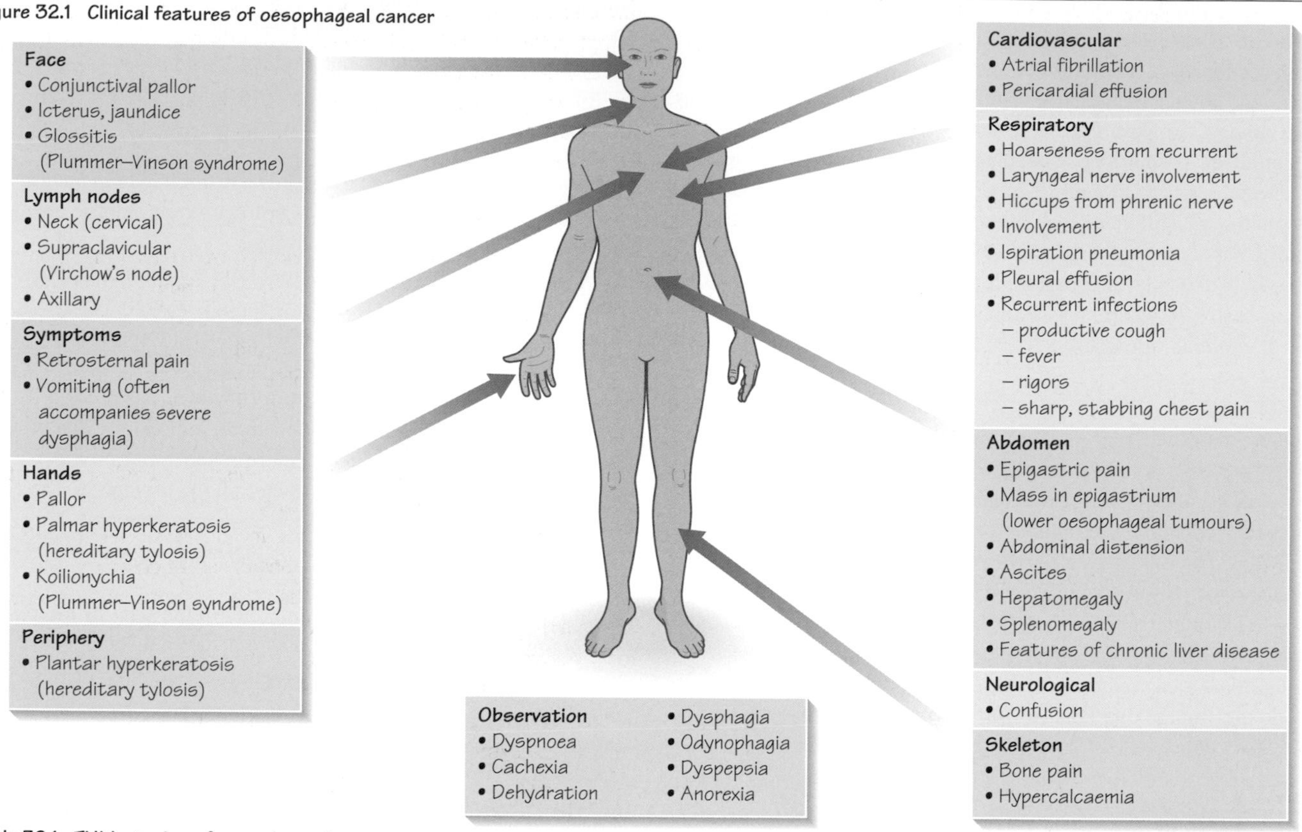

Face
- Conjunctival pallor
- Icterus, jaundice
- Glossitis
  (Plummer–Vinson syndrome)

Lymph nodes
- Neck (cervical)
- Supraclavicular
  (Virchow's node)
- Axillary

Symptoms
- Retrosternal pain
- Vomiting (often
  accompanies severe
  dysphagia)

Hands
- Pallor
- Palmar hyperkeratosis
  (hereditary tylosis)
- Koilionychia
  (Plummer–Vinson syndrome)

Periphery
- Plantar hyperkeratosis
  (hereditary tylosis)

Cardiovascular
- Atrial fibrillation
- Pericardial effusion

Respiratory
- Hoarseness from recurrent
- Laryngeal nerve involvement
- Hiccups from phrenic nerve
- Involvement
- Ispiration pneumonia
- Pleural effusion
- Recurrent infections
  – productive cough
  – fever
  – rigors
  – sharp, stabbing chest pain

Abdomen
- Epigastric pain
- Mass in epigastrium
  (lower oesophageal tumours)
- Abdominal distension
- Ascites
- Hepatomegaly
- Splenomegaly
- Features of chronic liver disease

Neurological
- Confusion

Skeleton
- Bone pain
- Hypercalcaemia

Observation
- Dyspnoea
- Cachexia
- Dehydration
- Dysphagia
- Odynophagia
- Dyspepsia
- Anorexia

Table 32.1 TNM staging of oesophageal cancer

Classification	Division	Description
T – extent of tumour	Tx	The primary tumour cannot be evaluated
	T0	There is no evidence of a primary tumour in the stomach
	Tis	Carcinoma in situ
	T1	Tumour invading into the lamina propria/submucosa
	T2	Tumour invading into the muscularis propria
	T3	Tumour has penetrated the adventitia
	T4a	Tumour has invaded into the pleura, the pericardium, or the diaphragm
	T4b	Tumour has spread into other nearby structures such as the trachea, vertebra, or the aorta.
N – regional lymph nodes	Nx	Regional lymph nodes cannot be evaluated
	N0	No regional lymphadenopathy
	N1	Regional lymph node involvement (one or two lymph nodes)
	N2	Regional lymph node involvement (three to six lymph nodes)
	N3	Regional lymph node involvement (seven or more lymph nodes)
M – metastasis	Mx	Distant metastasis cannot be evaluated
	M0	No distant metastasis
	M1	Distant metastasis

Epidemiology

Approximately 4000 people die each year from oesophageal cancer, making it the ninth most common cancer in adults in the UK. There are very few cases in people under the age of 45 and the incidence increases eightfold between 45–54 and 65–74 years. It has a sevenfold higher incidence in men than women. It is 20–30 times more common in China than in the USA.

Aetiology and pathophysiology

One-third of oesophageal cancers are adenocarcinoma, mostly found in the distal oesophagus. Two-thirds are squamous cell cancers with 15% in upper, 45% in mid and 40% in lower portions of the oesophagus.

Squamous cell cancer of the oesophagus is associated with chronic irritation, possibly caused by alcohol, caustic injury, radiotherapy or achalasia. The Plummer–Vinson syndrome (sideroblastic anaemia, glossitis, oesophagitis), chronic iron deficiency anaemia and dysphagia are associated with squamous cell cancers, particularly in impoverished populations. Hereditary tylosis, an autosomal dominant trait which causes palmar-plantar hyperkeratosis, carries a 95% risk of squamous cell cancer by the age of 70.

Adenocarcinoma is associated with gastro-oesophageal reflux, hiatus hernia, obesity and frequent antacid or histamine H2 blocker use. Barrett's oesophagus develops in 8% of patients with reflux, leading to metaplasia of the normal squamous epithelium of the lower oesophagus to columnar epithelium, which may be dysplastic, and the annual transformation to adenocarcinoma is 0.5%.

In recent years there has been a shift of diagnosis from squamous to adenocarcinoma, perhaps reflecting the changing patterns of smoking, obesity and nutrition of patients.

Rare tumours of the oesophagus include small cell carcinoma, mucoepidermoid carcinoma, sarcoma, adenoid cystic carcinoma and primary lymphoma.

Clinical presentation

Dysphagia is a common presenting symptom associated with weight loss and, rarely, haematemesis. The dysphagia can deteriorate rapidly over a period of weeks to months, typically progressive in nature and worse for solids than liquids. Other symptoms include dyspepsia, dyspnoea, odynophagia (advanced stages) and iron deficiency anaemia. Weight loss of >10% of total body weight is associated with a worse outcome.

The tumour may invade adjacent anatomical structures, leading to recurrent pneumonia or aspiration pneumonia due to an oesophageal fistula. Left supraclavicular lymphadenopathy (Virchow's node), hepatomegaly and pleural effusion are common features of advanced disease at presentation. Rapid exsanguination may occur if the tumour invades the thoracic aorta. Involvement of the pericardium is uncommon but can result in arrhythmia and pericardial effusions. Hoarseness may be a sign of recurrent laryngeal nerve involvement. Hiccups may be a sign of phrenic nerve involvement. Bone involvement can be identified by pain or associated hypercalcaemia

Investigations and staging

A diagnosis is usually confirmed by upper GI endoscopy and biopsy. Barium studies are an alternative for patients who cannot tolerate endoscopy but precludes biopsy. Laparoscopy may be useful for distal tumours. Endoscopic ultrasound is very accurate in determining the depth of invasion but less accurate in determining nodal involvement. CT imaging of the chest, abdomen and pelvis is required for staging the disease and determining the extent of spread and involvement of lymph nodes. PET-CT is increasingly used before surgery to determine the extent of disease and operability (Table 32.1). Bronchoscopy may be required to detect tracheal invasion. Bone scan imaging should be arranged if the patient complains of bone pain or has hypercalcaemia at presentation.

Treatment

Surgical resection, sometimes with neoadjuvant chemotherapy (cisplatin, carboplatin, or oxaliplatin with fluorouracil and epirubicin) or chemoradiation, is the treatment of choice for early stage oesophageal cancer but many patients have precluding surgical co-morbidities such that <40% of patients are suitable for resection with oesophagectomy. Operative mortality is approximately 5–10% and complications include anastomotic leakage, strictures, reflux and motility problems. The role and benefit of adjuvant chemotherapy is unclear and patients should be considered for clinical trials.

At diagnosis, 25% have locally advanced disease. Those with small volume inoperable disease may be considered for chemoradiation with curative intent, but this can cause oesophageal perforation or stricture, pneumonitis and pulmonary fibrosis. The majority of patients with locally advanced disease are treated with stent insertion for dysphagia or palliative radiotherapy for pain or bleeding.

The remaining patients (35%) present with metastatic disease and are treated symptomatically or with palliative combination chemotherapy (as above) if sufficiently fit. Some patients may be considered for palliative radiotherapy with brachytherapy in some patients. Laser treatment and stent insertion can restore the oesophageal lumen and relieve dysphagia.

Prognosis

The survival of oesophageal cancer correlates with stage at presentation. Patients with in situ disease have a >95% 5-year survival, but this falls to 30–80% for local disease, 10–30% with nodal involvement and <2% with metastatic disease.

Approximately 25% of patients are suitable for surgical resection, producing a 5-year survival of 25%. Overall, considering all patients from diagnosis, the 5-year survival in the UK is 8%.

Half of all oesophageal cancer could be prevented by education about smoking cessation, drinking less alcohol, improving diet with more fresh fruit and vegetables, and reducing poorly preserved and high salt foods.

Endoscopic surveillance is required for 2–5 years for patients with Barrett's oesophagus. Low-grade dysplasia requires proton-pump inhibitor therapy, while high-grade dysplasia requires surgical resection.

Figure 33.1 Clinical features of gastric cancer

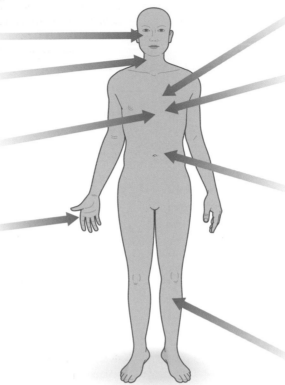

Face
- Conjunctival pallor
- Icterus, jaundice

Lymph nodes
- Neck (cervical)
- Supraclavicular (Virchow's node)
- Axillary (particularly left)

Symptoms
- Retrosternal pain
- Dyspepsia
- Dysphagia
- Nausea and vomiting

Hands
- Pallor
- Palmar hyperkeratosis
  (hereditary tylosis)
- Koilionychia
  (Plummer–Vinson syndrome)

Observation
- Cachexia
- Dehydration
- Anorexia
- Dermatomyositis
- Acanthosis nigricans

Cardiovascular
– (all rare)
- Atrial fibrillation
- Pericardial effusion

Respiratory
- Pleural effusion

Abdomen
- Epigastric pain
- Mass in epigastrium
- Abdominal distension
- Ascites
- Melaena
- Hepatomegaly
- Pelvic mass
  (Krukenberg tumour)
- Metastasis to ovary
- Umbilical nodule
  (Sister Mary Joseph nodule)
- Metastatic rectal shelf
- Palpable PR (Blumer's shelf)

Neurological
- Confusion
- Carcinomatous meningitis

Skeleton
- Bone pain
- Hypercalcaemia

Table 33.1 TNM staging of gastric cancer

Classification	Division	Description
	Tx	The primary tumour cannot be evaluated
	T0	There is no evidence of a primary tumour in the stomach
	Tis	Carcinoma in situ
T – extent of tumour	T1	Tumour invading into the lamina propria/submucosa
	T2	Tumour invading into the muscularis propria/suberosa
	T3	Tumour has penetrated the serosa
	T4	Tumour has invaded organs surrounding the stomach
	Nx	Regional lymph nodes cannot be evaluated
	N0	No regional lymphadenopathy
N – regional lymph nodes	N1	Regional lymph node involvement (one or two lymph nodes)
	N2	Regional lymph node involvement (seven to 15 lymph nodes)
	N3	Regional lymph node involvement (16 or more lymph nodes)
	Mx	Distant metastasis cannot be evaluated
M – metastasis	M0	No distant metastasis
	M1	Distant metastasis

Epidemiology

Gastric cancer is the sixth most common cancer in the UK, accounting for 5% of all cancers. Worldwide it is the second most common cancer. The male:female ratio is around 1.8:1 and 95% of cases are diagnosed in people aged 55 or older, with an average age at presentation of 65 years.

The incidence of gastric cancer has fallen in the developed world, possibly due to better food preservation. It is more common in people with blood group A (20% increased risk). There are extreme variations by geographical location, 40% of cases occur in China, where it is the most common cancer, but age-adjusted incidence rates are highest in Japan with diet as the main contributing factor.

Aetiology

Dietary carcinogens can contribute to an increased risk of gastric cancer, especially nitrosamines and a diet high in salty foods (e.g. in Japan). *Helicobacter pylori* has been used to explain the aetiology of cancers developing in patients with atrophic gastritis as it is more common in patients with gastric cancer than without. Furthermore, chronic atrophic gastritis leads to a decrease in acid secretion with resulting bacterial overgrowth and an increase in nitrates. This is associated with a threefold increase in risk of gastric cancer. Familial mutations of cadherin-1 gene (*CDH1*) are associated with an increased risk. The routine use of proton-pump inhibitors without investigation with endoscopy may contribute to late diagnosis. Vagotomy and partial gastrectomy (20 years after surgery) carry an increased risk of gastric cancer. Other risk factors include family history, obesity, radiation and a lower socioeconomic class.

Pathophysiology

More than 95% of gastric cancers are adenocarcinoma and can be further categorised into intestinal and diffuse adenocarcinoma. Intestinal adenocarcinoma has a better prognosis and is associated with older patients, occurring more commonly in the distal stomach. Diffuse adenocarcinoma is more common and has a worse prognosis. Other rare tumours include squamous cell carcinoma (4%), lymphoma, gastrointestinal stromal tumours (GIST) and neuroendocrine tumours.

Clinical presentation

Early stage stomach cancer may be symptomless or have vague and non-specific symptoms (e.g. dyspepsia, tiredness or anorexia). Most patients will present with vague epigastric discomfort, which is worse with meals, weight loss, early satiety, anorexia, dysphagia, or vomiting. Features of advanced disease include ascites, jaundice, melaena, hepatomegaly (25% of patients have liver metastasis) and lymph node involvement (Virchow's node in the left SCF can be palpated in 33% of patients at presentation and half of patients have a palpable epigastric mass). Transcoelomic spread to the ovaries (Krukenberg tumour) is a rare complication.

Investigations and staging

Referral to a specialist for urgent endoscopy and review is required for patients >55 years presenting with dyspepsia alone or for patients <55 years presenting with dysphagia, vomiting, anorexia, weight loss or symptoms associated with gastrointestinal bleeding (e.g. breathlessness, tiredness).

Full blood count may show a microcytic anaemia due to blood loss and iron deficiency. Liver function tests may be abnormal due to liver metastasis. See Chapter 15 for discussion on serum tumour markers.

Endoscopy with biopsy is essential and if gastric ulceration is noted, a repeat endoscopy is required to confirm healing. A non-healing ulcer may suggest the possibility of malignancy. Barium studies may be helpful in those patients intolerant of endoscopy but preclude a biopsy for histological examination.

Ultrasound scanning of the liver and chest X-ray are useful tests to screen for metastasis, but many patients with advanced disease will require additional imaging. CT imaging of the thorax and abdomen can demonstrate involvement of local lymph nodes and identify metastasis (Table 33.1). PET imaging is increasing in use for the detection of disease spread.

Treatment

Surgery with laparotomy is the only significant curative intervention, often preceded with laparoscopic staging. However, only 50% of patients are suitable for surgery. Surgical developments have been driven by the Japanese and there is debate about the optimal surgery. For antral cancers, a subtotal gastrectomy has fewer complications compared with a total gastrectomy. Extensive lymphadenectomy, removing lymph nodes along the coeliac axis, hepatic and splenic arteries, allows more accurate staging and appears to improve survival. Patients with mid-gastric tumours require a total gastrectomy, whereas tumours of the gastro-oesophageal junction require subtotal resection of the oesophagus in addition to the cardia and gastric fundus.

For early-stage disease, endoscopic mucosal resection can be curative, with significantly reduced morbidity.

There are high relapse rates following surgery and unfortunately the benefits of adjuvant chemotherapy have not been as great as hoped. Patients should be considered for clinical trials, which are evaluating new schedules and agents. Adjuvant radiotherapy reduces locoregional relapse but does not alter survival.

Patients with locally advanced disease may become operable following neoadjuvant chemotherapy or chemoradiation.

Metastatic disease may be treated with fluoropyrimidine-based combination chemotherapy schedules. These have response rates of about 35% but do not significantly improve survival. Such patients are considered for clinical trials of new targeted agents and biological therapies. Patients who have HER2 overexpressing metastatic gastric or gastro-oesophageal junction adenocarcinoma, and who have not received prior treatment for their metastatic disease, can be treated with trastuzumab in combination with cisplatin and a fluoropyrimidine. Other palliative approaches may be required to improve symptoms. Endoscopic laser treatment can be used to reduce bleeding from intraluminal tumours, rigid or expandable metal stents can relieve dysphagia due to tumours of the oesophagogastric junction and cardia of the stomach.

Prognosis

More than 50% of patients in the UK present with advanced disease and therefore the 5-year survival is around 15%. In patients under 50 years, the 5-year survival is 16–22% compared with 5–12% in those over 70. For patients with advanced local disease at presentation or metastatic disease, the median survival is approximately 6 months.

Figure 34.1 Clinical features of colorectal cancer

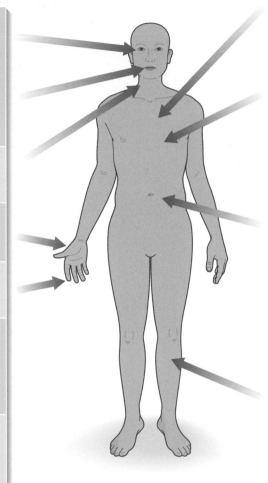

Face
- Eyes
  - conjunctival pallor (IDA)
  - corneal arcus (hyperlipidaemia)
  - xanthelasma (hyperlipidaemia)
  - jaundice of sclera (liver involvement)
- Mouth
  - mucosal pallor (IDA)
  - angular cheilitis (IDA)
  - atrophic glossitis (IDA)

Lymph nodes
- Troisier's sign
  (enlarged Virchow's lymph
  node in the left SCF)

Hands
- Palmar xanthoma
  (hyperlipidaemia)
- Dupuytrens contractures

Nails
- Clubbing (ulcerative colitis)
- Tar staining (smoking)
- Koilonychia (IDA)

Observation
- Cachexia
- Obesity
- Writhing
  - colicky abdominal pain
- Skin
  - erythema gyratum repens

Abbreviations
- IDA
  - iron deficiency anaemia
- FAP
  - familial adenomatous polyposis

Cardiovascular
- Iron deficiency anaemia
  - tachycardia
  - flow murmur
  - cardiac enlargement
  - ankle oedema
  - heart failure

Respiratory
- Lung involvement
  - cough
  - dysponea
  - chest pain
  - haemoptysis
  - pleural effusion
  - wheeze/stridor
  - SVC obstruction
  - Horner's syndrome

Abdomen
- Surgical scars
- Abdominal distension
- Stoma
- Fistula
  - colovesical (faecal debris in the urine)
  - colovaginal (leakage of faeces PV)
  - ischiorectal/perineal abscesses
- Peritoneal involvement
  - ascites
- Liver involvement
  - hepatomegaly
  - jaundice

Skeletal survey
- Bone involvement
- Focal bone tenderness

Specific FAP extracolonic features
- Congenital hypertrophy of the
  retinal pigment epithelium (CHRPE)
- Osteomas of the jaw
- Pre-pubertal epidermoid cysts

Table 34.1 TNM staging of colorectal cancer

Classification	Division	Description
	T0	No evidence of primary tumour
	T1	Tumour invading submucosa
T – extent of tumour	T2	Tumour invading muscularis
	T3	Tumour invading through muscularis
	T4	Tumour perforating the peritoneum
	N0	No nodal involvement
	N1	Metastasis in one to three pericolic nodes
N – regional lymph nodes	N2	Metastasis in four or more pericolic nodes
	N3	Lymph node involvement on named vascular trunk or apical node metastasis in any lymph nodes
M – metastasis	M0	No distant metastasis
	M1	Distant metastasis

Epidemiology

Colorectal cancer is the third most common cancer and second most common cause of cancer death in the UK. Occurrence is strongly related to age, with almost 85% of cases occurring in people aged 60 years and over. It is significantly more common in the developed world, occurring most frequently in New Zealand, Canada, USA and UK. There is no gender bias.

Aetiology

Colorectal cancer is generally considered to be an environmental disease, with the majority of cases being linked to lifestyle and advancing age, and only a minority occurring as a result of genetic predisposition.

Many of the lifestyle factors thought to encourage development of colorectal adenocarcinoma are diet-related and increased consumption of red meat, alcohol and a high calorie intake play an important role. Other risk factors include smoking, sedentary lifestyle and obesity. Colorectal cancer occurs more commonly in patients with inflammatory bowel disease and risk increases with duration of disease and severity of bowel inflammation.

Approximately 5% of all colorectal cancer cases occur as a consequence of genetic syndromes, the most common of which is hereditary non-polyposis colorectal cancer (HNPCC or Lynch syndrome type I). HNPCC develops as a consequence of germ-line mutations in one of several DNA mismatch repair genes and carries a 40% lifetime risk of developing colorectal cancer. The condition is transmitted in an autosomal dominant pattern. Patients with HNPCC typically develop colorectal cancer in the fourth decade of life. Other malignancies such as ovarian, endometrial, gastric, urinary and hepatobiliary cancer may occur and these are recognised as Lynch syndrome type II (see Chapter 8).

Familial adenomatous polyposis (FAP) is a more rare type of hereditary colorectal cancer. It is inherited in an autosomal dominant pattern and arises as a result of germ-line mutations in the tumour suppressor gene *APC*. From a young age, affected patients develop numerous benign colonic polyps, which will eventually transform into cancerous lesions, typically in the third and fourth decades of life. Prophylactic colectomy is therefore strongly advised.

Pathophysiology

More than 70% of all colorectal cancers are adenocarcinomas arising in the mucosa from benign adenomatous polyps. Adenomas are typically slow growing, with a minority progressing to malignancy if they are not surgically removed. This risk of malignant transformation is increased with increasing size of the adenoma and with the length of time it has been present. Once a tumour has become established, it can spread through the layers of the bowel wall and may eventually metastasise to the liver, lungs, bone, brain and skin. Several genetic alterations have been implicated in the progression of benign adenomas to invasive adenocarcinomas.

Clinical presentation

In its early stages, colorectal cancer is often asymptomatic and hence 55% of patients present with advanced disease. Patients with right-sided cancer typically present with a palpable mass in the right iliac fossa, diarrhoea, weight loss, anaemia and occult gastrointestinal bleeding. The clinical features of a left-sided cancer include a palpable mass in the left iliac fossa, change in bowel habit (most commonly constipation), tenesmus, rectal bleeding, and signs and symptoms of bowel obstruction. Patients with left-sided cancer typically present earlier than those with right-sided cancer.

Investigations and staging

All patients with suspected colorectal cancer require rectal examination, full blood count, and assessment of renal and liver function. Colonoscopy should be performed and, if patients are unsuitable for colonoscopy, a flexible sigmoidoscopy and double contrast barium enema is an alternative. CT imaging of chest, abdomen and pelvis is helpful to determine the extent of the disease and may aid assessment of operability. Carcinoembryonic antigen (CEA) may be elevated and is useful for assessing response to treatment. The TNM staging system is commonly used (Table 34.1) and the Duke's stage reflects the degree of invasion:

- Duke's stage A: tumour confined to mucosa;
- Duke's stage B: tumour has breached the serosa;
- Duke's stage C: regional lymph nodes are involved;
- Duke's stage D: distant metastases are present.

Treatment

Surgery should be considered for most patients to mobilise and remove the tumour and remove regional lymph nodes. Liver metastasis can be considered for resection. Eighty per cent of all tumours are resectable and most are treated by hemicolectomy. Rectal surgery is more challenging, but advances in total mesorectal excision have led to an improvement in survival.

Radiotherapy has little impact on survival in rectal cancer but it can be used as neoadjuvant treatment in rectal cancer, to shrink the tumour before surgery and limit pelvic recurrence.

Half of all patients treated with curative intent resection are likely to relapse within 2 years of surgery. Adjuvant chemotherapy using 5-fluorouracil and irinotecan regimens has improved survival for both colon and rectal cancers.

Biological therapies that target vascular endothelial growth factor (bevacizumab) and the epidermal growth factor receptor (cetuximab) have produced real improvements in outcome for patients with advanced or metastatic disease.

Prognosis

The 5-year survival for colorectal cancer by Duke's stage is: A, 93%; B, 77%; C, 48%; and D, 7%.

Screening

Four randomised controlled studies have shown that population screening of people over age 50 years for faecal occult blood reduces colorectal cancer deaths. A pilot screening programme is underway in the UK. Patients with abnormal results will be referred for colonoscopic investigation and it is estimated that this may reduce mortality by up to 16%. One-off flexible sigmoidoscopy screening to men and women aged 55–59 years has been reported to be effective. High-risk patient groups such as those with HNPCC and FAP or those with a longstanding diagnosis of ulcerative colitis will require regular surveillance with colonoscopy.

Figure 35.1 Clinical features of pancreatic cancer

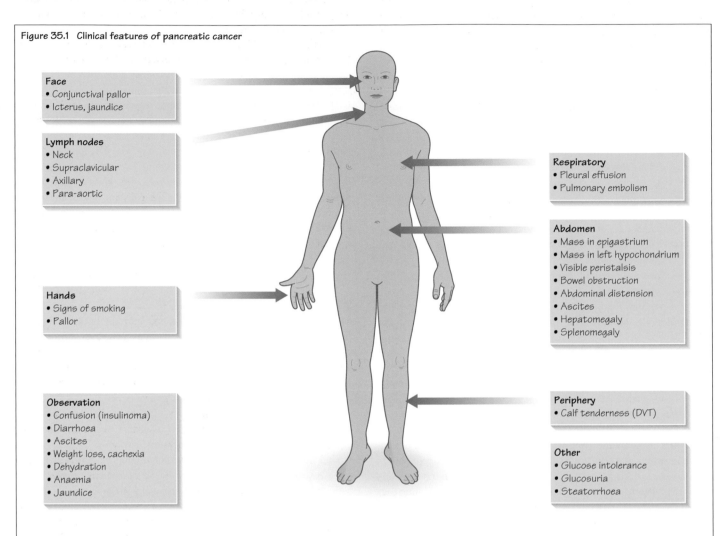

Face
- Conjunctival pallor
- Icterus, jaundice

Lymph nodes
- Neck
- Supraclavicular
- Axillary
- Para-aortic

Hands
- Signs of smoking
- Pallor

Observation
- Confusion (insulinoma)
- Diarrhoea
- Ascites
- Weight loss, cachexia
- Dehydration
- Anaemia
- Jaundice

Respiratory
- Pleural effusion
- Pulmonary embolism

Abdomen
- Mass in epigastrium
- Mass in left hypochondrium
- Visible peristalsis
- Bowel obstruction
- Abdominal distension
- Ascites
- Hepatomegaly
- Splenomegaly

Periphery
- Calf tenderness (DVT)

Other
- Glucose intolerance
- Glucosuria
- Steatorrhoea

Table 35.1 TNM staging of pancreatic cancer

Classification	Division	Description
T – extent of tumour	Tis	Carcinoma in situ (very few tumours are found at this stage)
	T1	Tumour has not spread beyond the pancreas and is smaller than 2 cm
	T2	Tumour has not spread beyond the pancreas but is larger than 2 cm
	T3	Tumour has spread from the pancreas to surrounding tissues near the pancreas but not to major blood vessels or nerves
	T4	Tumour has extended beyond the pancreas and invades nearby large blood vessels or nerves
N – regional lymph nodes	N0	Regional lymph nodes are not involved
	N1	Regional lymph nodes are involved with tumour
M – metastasis	M0	Tumour has not spread to distant lymph nodes (other than those near the pancreas) or to distant organs such as the liver, lungs, or brain
	M1	Distant metastasis is present

Epidemiology

Pancreatic cancer is the tenth most common cancer in the UK, with approximately 7600 diagnoses made each year, and the fifth most common cause of cancer death. The average age of diagnosis is between 60 and 65, but 40% present below the age of 75. It is more common in males until age 75, above which incidence in women is higher.

Aetiology

Smoking is the only well-established aetiological factor in pancreatic cancer with a fivefold increase in risk; studies of alcohol and coffee consumption have been contradictory. Some studies have identified diabetes mellitus and chronic pancreatitis as risk factors; however, as both may develop as a consequence of pancreatic cancer the results have been questioned.

Over 90% are adenocarcinoma of ductal origin, 5% are endocrine tumours arising in islet cells and 5% are acinar cell tumours.

Clinical presentation

Two-thirds of pancreatic cancers occur in the head of pancreas, and patients present with epigastric pain, weight loss and jaundice. The remaining third of tumours occur in the body and tail of pancreas and cause pain in the left upper quadrant of the abdomen with constipation due to colonic involvement. The pain increases in severity over time and radiates to the back, coinciding with retroperitoneal invasion. This pain characteristically improves when the patient leans forward. Tumours in the tail and body tend to be larger at the time of diagnosis and therefore have a worse prognosis.

Occasionally tumours are periampullary and cause obstructive jaundice at an early stage. This can result in an earlier diagnosis and therefore these tumours have a better outcome.

Tumours may extend directly into the duodenum, stomach and retroperitoneum. Tumours that present late often have involvement of the locoregional lymph nodes, particularly portal and para-aortic. Metastases may be present at diagnosis, and the liver and lung are common sites. Many patients are asymptomatic until the common bile duct becomes blocked and they become jaundiced. Rarely, splenomegaly and varices can result from splenic vein occlusion by a tumour in the body or tail of pancreas.

Diabetes mellitus may be the presenting feature of pancreatic malignancy months before any other signs or symptoms emerge. Other presenting features include Trousseau sign of malignancy (superficial migratory thrombophlebitis), fever caused by cholangitis and ascites due to peritoneal involvement.

Investigations and staging

Early pancreatic cancer is difficult to diagnose, but should be considered in any individual with ongoing upper abdominal pain. Investigation is aimed at establishing the prognosis and defining operability.

Endoluminal ultrasound can produce clearer images than abdominal ultrasound as the probe is passed down the oesophagus and achieves a closer proximity to the pancreas. CT imaging can reveal a mass, evidence of invasion and lymph node involvement, or metastasis. Endoscopic retrograde cholangiopancreatography (ERCP) is required and during the procedure, brushings, suction of the pancreatic duct, or biopsy can be performed. A stent can be inserted during the initial procedure. Failure to obtain a diagnosis should be followed by an image-guided biopsy by FNA or rarely a laparoscopic biopsy or assessment prior to surgery.

Blood tests for full blood count, renal and liver function, and serum CA19-9 tumour marker should be arranged (see Chapter 15).

Staging

The TNM staging system is used, but practically, pancreatic cancer can be grouped by whether it is resectable, locally advanced (non-resectable), or metastatic at presentation (Table 35.1).

Treatment

One-third of patients present with pancreatic cancer so advanced that the only treatment options available are pain relief and symptom control. Most patients are treated symptomatically with endoscopic stenting for jaundice, occasionally surgical gastric bypass for duodenal obstruction and coeliac plexus nerve block for pain.

Surgery is the only treatment option that offers the possibility of long-term remission, but pancreaticoduodenectomy and total pancreatectomy are major procedures with high complication rates and serious morbidity. Surgical feasibility depends on the tumour size, spread and overall performance status of the patient. Only about 20% of cases meet these criteria, and cure will be an outcome for a small minority. At laparotomy, only 30% of patients with radiologically operable tumours actually have surgically operable disease. For some patients surgical resection is beneficial for symptom improvement. Others with more advanced disease may be suitable for biliary stenting or bypass procedures. Complications of the surgery can be significant with some patients becoming diabetic and losing pancreatic exocrine function, requiring the use of pancreatic enzymes and insulin.

Radiotherapy is most useful in those with locally advanced disease for palliation of pain in particular. The radiation dose required is high, at 40–60 Gy, so adverse effects may outweigh benefits.

Chemotherapy may be used for palliation. Pancreatic cancer is resistant to most chemotherapy agents but gemcitabine, a nucleoside analogue, has been shown to improve both symptom and disease control. Chemotherapy can be administered before or after surgery, in advanced disease and in combination with radiotherapy. A chemotherapy combination, FOLFIRINOX (5-fluorouracil, folinic acid, irinotecan, and oxaliplatin), has been shown in clinical trials to provide a better survival time in advanced pancreatic cancer than gemcitabine alone, but is considerably more toxic.

Prognosis

The prognosis of pancreatic cancer is notoriously poor but improvements in palliative care have led to a modest increase in short-term survival. For patients with locally advanced or metastatic disease the median survival is 3–4 months. For those that have had surgical resection the median survival is 11–20 months.

The 1-year survival is approximately 16% and 5-year survival is very low at about 3%. Patients diagnosed early with periampullary cancer have a better prognosis, with 5-year survival of up to 50%.

Figure 36.1   Clinical features of hepatobiliary cancer

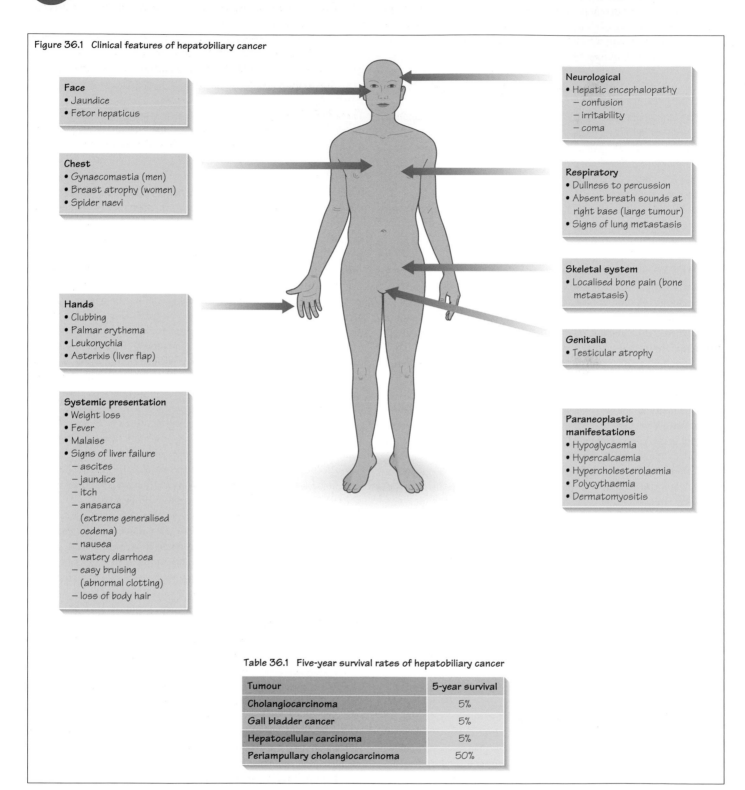

Face
• Jaundice
• Fetor hepaticus

Neurological
• Hepatic encephalopathy
  – confusion
  – irritability
  – coma

Chest
• Gynaecomastia (men)
• Breast atrophy (women)
• Spider naevi

Respiratory
• Dullness to percussion
• Absent breath sounds at right base (large tumour)
• Signs of lung metastasis

Skeletal system
• Localised bone pain (bone metastasis)

Hands
• Clubbing
• Palmar erythema
• Leukonychia
• Asterixis (liver flap)

Genitalia
• Testicular atrophy

Systemic presentation
• Weight loss
• Fever
• Malaise
• Signs of liver failure
  – ascites
  – jaundice
  – itch
  – anasarca
    (extreme generalised oedema)
  – nausea
  – watery diarrhoea
  – easy bruising
    (abnormal clotting)
  – loss of body hair

Paraneoplastic manifestations
• Hypoglycaemia
• Hypercalcaemia
• Hypercholesterolaemia
• Polycythaemia
• Dermatomyositis

Table 36.1   Five-year survival rates of hepatobiliary cancer

Tumour	5-year survival
Cholangiocarcinoma	5%
Gall bladder cancer	5%
Hepatocellular carcinoma	5%
Periampullary cholangiocarcinoma	50%

Epidemiology

Hepatocellular carcinoma (HCC) is one of the most common cancers worldwide, but is less common in the UK with approximately 2800 cases per year (1% of all cancer diagnoses and 40% of hepatobiliary cancers). The distribution of HCC closely aligns with that of chronic HBV infection, with most cases in East Asia and Sub-Saharan Africa. HCC is four to eight times more common in men than in women and most diagnoses are made during the fifth or sixth decade of life, corresponding with time taken for liver cirrhosis to develop.

Secondary metastases to the liver, rather than primary liver tumours, are more common in the UK, particularly from primaries in the colon, pancreas, stomach, breast and lung.

Cholangiocarcinoma (usually adenocarcinoma) accounts for more than 50% of hepatobiliary cancer in the UK, affecting the bile ducts inside or outside the liver. It is a relatively rare cancer with around 1000 cases per year in the UK. Other rarer types of hepatobiliary cancer include angiosarcoma and hepatoblastoma, a cancer affecting children under 3 years.

Aetiology

More than 70% of HCC cases worldwide are associated with chronic infection with hepatitis B or C viruses. The lifetime risk of developing HCC is 40% in HBV-infected individuals and is thought to be higher for HCV infection. Other risk factors include alcoholic cirrhosis, aflatoxin (a fungal contaminant of crops in tropical regions), primary biliary cirrhosis and inherited metabolic disorders such as haemochromatosis and tyrosinaemia.

Individuals with primary sclerosing cholangitis have a lifetime risk of developing cholangiocarcinoma of 10–20%. Infection with liver flukes has been implicated and accounts for the higher prevalence of cholangiocarcinoma in Southeast Asia.

Clinical presentation

Early stage HCC is often asymptomatic or with vague symptoms including weight loss, nausea and lethargy. There may be abdominal pain in the right upper quadrant due to stretching of the liver capsule. There can be referred pain to the right shoulder as the enlarging liver irritates the diaphragm. If the tumour obstructs a bile duct, then HCC may present with features of obstructive jaundice.

Late presenting features are those of liver failure, depending on the functional reserve of the liver (often depleted in those with cirrhosis). Acute onset abdominal pain and distension are features of intraperitoneal haemorrhage, which can be life threatening.

Cholangiocarcinoma tends to present with jaundice, pruritis and hepatomegaly as early features. Later signs and symptoms include right upper quadrant pain, weight loss and a palpable gall bladder (Courvoisier's sign).

Investigations and staging

Initial investigations should include full blood count, liver and renal function, chest X-ray and ultrasound assessment of the liver. A lesion identified in a cirrhotic liver is often HCC. The serum tumour marker alpha-fetoprotein (AFP) is elevated in 75% of cases, and the combination of an ultrasound lesion >2 cm and raised AFP are diagnostic. Other tumour markers such as CEA and CA19-9 may be useful for monitoring the disease (see Chapter 15).

CT imaging can determine the extent of spread but MRI with contrast and angiography provides the detail required to inform the most effective treatment. Liver biopsy may be necessary but risks seeding tumour cells outside the liver.

In cholangiocarcinoma the liver function tests often show a raised conjugated bilirubin and elevation of serum CEA and CA19-9. Ultrasound imaging will reveal the level of obstruction and MRI cholangiography (MRCP) provides a clear picture of the biliary tree.

Treatment

Surgery offers the only chance of cure for HCC but is only possible in a minority of patients, as success is limited by background cirrhosis. In an otherwise healthy liver, it is possible to resect up to 80% and it will regenerate. However, even a small resection can induce liver failure in a cirrhotic patient. Liver transplant is the preferred treatment for those with cirrhosis, although only for tumours <3 cm. It is preferred for those with HCV as it is likely HCC will recur in these patients.

When surgical resection is not possible, sclerotherapy or hepatic embolisation can be considered, where chemotherapy agents are injected into the hepatic artery for local effect and an embolising agent is injected to cut off the blood supply to the tumour. Radiofrequency ablation can be used to induce tumour necrosis and is best for more superficial lesions.

Chemotherapy may be more appropriate in advanced disease and agents such as mitoxantrone, gemcitabine and doxorubicin have been used, but the cancer is relatively resistant to most agents. A receptor tyrosine kinase inhibitor, sorafenib, inhibits tumour cell proliferation and angiogenesis, producing a median overall survival of 9.2 months and median time to progression of 5.5 months.

Stenting of the biliary tree is required for those patients with obstructive jaundice.

If cholangiocarcinoma is detected in its early stages, the bile ducts can be resected, but these tumours tend to present late when symptoms appear. If the cancer has spread to the liver it can still be resected or a Whipple's procedure performed, where part of the stomach, duodenum, pancreas and gall bladder are removed. If surgery is not possible, a stent can be inserted to allow bile to flow past the obstruction. Tumours of the biliary tree are often very sensitive to chemotherapy, with gemcitabine and cisplatin producing benefit in cholangiocarcinoma.

Prognosis

The overall 5-year survival rate for patients with operable liver cancer is approximately 30%, when management involves a partial liver resection. For patients receiving a liver transplant the 5-year survival is 75%. The median survival of patients not considered for curative therapy is 6–7 months with 5% of patients alive at 5 years after diagnosis.

Cholangiocarcinoma has a 5% 5-year survival. The worst prognosis is with intrahepatic cholangiocarcinoma, which has a median survival is 12–18 months from diagnosis (Table 36.1).

It is important to consider that the most important intervention for hepatocellular carcinoma is the development of an effective vaccination programme against hepatitis B, particularly in geographical locations where the virus is endemic.

37 Ovarian cancer

Figure 37.1 Clinical features of ovarian cancer

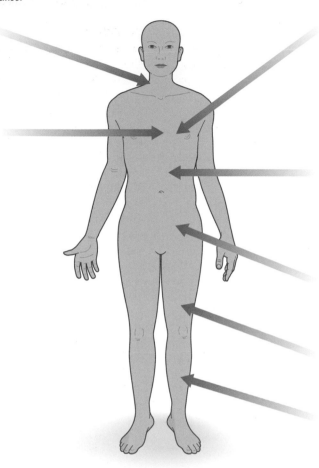

Lymph nodes
- Neck
- Supraclavicular
- Axillary
- Inguinal
- Para-aortic

Cardiovascular
- Pericardial effusion
- Loud P2 (pulmonary hypertension, PE)

Observation
- Virilisation (Sertoli–Leydig)
- Ascites
- Skin
  - dermatomyositis
  - cachexia
  - dehydration
  - nausea and vomiting

Other
- Haematuria
- PV discharge/bleeding
- PR examination
- PV examination

Respiratory
- Pleural effusion
- Pleural rub (PE)
- Tachypnoea (PE)

Abdomen
- Surgical scars
- Umbilical nodule
- Visible peristalsis
- Bowel obstruction
- Abdominal distension
- Ascites
- Hepatomegaly
- Hepatic tenderness
- Renal tenderness (hydroureter)
- Pelvic mass
- Adenexal mass

Neurological
- Focal neurological signs (rare)
- Cerebellar dysfunction (paraneoplastic)

Skeletal survey
- Focal bone tenderness (rare) (pelvis, spine, long bones)

Periphery
- Calf tenderness (DVT)

Table 37.1 FIGO staging of ovarian cancer

Stage	Description
1a	Tumour confined to one ovary
1b	Tumour involving both ovaries but no serosal involvement
1c	Tumour on the ovarian surface, capsular breach or rupture, or malignant ascites
2a	The tumour has extended and/or implanted into the uterus and/or the fallopian tubes. Malignant cells are not detected in ascites or peritoneal washings
2b	The tumour has extended to another organ in the pelvis. Malignant cells are not detected in ascites or peritoneal washings
2c	Tumours that are stage **2a** or **b** but malignant cells are detected in the ascites or peritoneal washings
3a	Microscopic peritoneal metastasis beyond the pelvis. No lymph node involvement
3b	Macroscopic peritoneal metastasis beyond the pelvis but <2 cm in greatest dimension
3c	Macroscopic peritoneal metastasis beyond the pelvis >2 cm in greatest dimension and/or regional lymph nodes metastasis
4	Distant metastasis or parenchymal liver or other visceral metastasis, malignant pleural effusion

Epidemiology

Ovarian cancer is the fourth most common cancer in the UK, accounting for 5% of all deaths in women aged 40–60 years. The average age at presentation is 60 years. Fallopian tube and peritoneal cancer can share histological features with ovarian cancer and are treated in a similar approach.

Aetiology

Suppressed ovulation appears to protect against the development of ovarian cancer, so pregnancy, prolonged breastfeeding and the high-oestrogen contraceptive pill have all been shown to reduce the risk of ovarian cancer.

Up to 7% of women with ovarian cancer have a positive family history. Patients with Peutz–Jeghers syndrome have a 10% risk of ovarian cancer. Two well-recognised familial patterns occur:
- hereditary breast/ovarian cancer families, which have mutations in the BRCA1 or BRCA2 gene;
- Lynch type II families, which have an increased risk of ovarian, endometrial, colorectal and gastric tumours and carry mutations in mismatch repair enzymes (see Chapter 8).

Pathophysiology

Epithelial tumours are the most common cancer of the ovary (90%). They include adenocarcinoma, which can have a variety of histological appearances including serous (46%), mucinous (36%), endometrioid (8%), clear cell (3%) and squamous cell carcinomas (<1%).

Other rare types of ovarian tumours include:
- germ cell tumours, which resemble testicular germ cell tumours in histology and clinical management (see Chapter 40);
- carcinosarcomas, which are aggressive and more susceptible to haematogenous spread;
- sex cord tumours, including granulosa cell tumours, thecomas, Sertoli–Leydig cell tumours and gonadoblastomas. These occasionally produce oestrogens, causing precocious puberty and postmenopausal bleeding, and androgens causing virilisation.

Clinical presentation

Early stage ovarian cancer is asymptomatic in the majority of cases. Therefore, most women present with advanced disease where symptoms of vague abdominal discomfort, bloating, altered bowel habit, nausea and vomiting, backache, or weight loss are more common. In fact, 70% of women present with advanced disease that is stage 3–4. Vaginal bleeding is uncommon but more likely in Fallopian tube cancer. It is important to consider and exclude ovarian cancer in women presenting with recent change in bowel habit or vague abdominal symptoms, such as those described in irritable bowel syndrome.

Pleural effusions, ascites, malignant bowel obstruction and thromboembolic phenomenon are all associated with more advanced disease. Occasionally, umbilical peritoneal deposits are seen as Sister Mary Joseph nodules indicating transcoelomic spread and stage 4 disease.

Investigation and staging

The combination of transvaginal ultrasound findings, serum CA125 and age can be used to differentiate between benign ovarian cysts and ovarian malignancy, with 80–90% sensitivity and specificity. These investigations have been studied for population screening (see Chapter 16). CT imaging may be useful to detect abdominal spread, including liver, lung, pleura and lymph node involvement. The staging and determination of extent of spread is determined with surgery and the FIGO staging system is outlined in Table 37.1.

Treatment

Surgery remains the first intervention for patients with ovarian cancer, with the intention of best effort debulking of the disease to achieve complete (no macroscopic disease), optimal (macroscopic disease <1 cm) or suboptimal debulking (residual disease >1 cm). Surgery involves a laparotomy, total hysterectomy, bilateral salpingo-oopherectomy with omentectomy and lymph node resection.

Following surgery the majority of women will be candidates for adjuvant chemotherapy with carboplatin and paclitaxel, but the addition of bevacizumab for those with high-risk disease is advantageous. Neoadjuvant chemotherapy is used for patients with extensive disease at presentation, with the aim of shrinking the disease in order to consider interval debulking. Non-epithelial ovarian cancer requires surgery followed by chemotherapy, based on the predominant cell type present. From diagnosis, 80% of patients achieve remission, 15% have residual disease and 5% progress on chemotherapy.

At relapse, second-line chemotherapy is associated with a response rate of 20–40%, with higher rates correlating with greater treatment-free intervals. Serum CA125 may be useful in predicting relapse (median 4.2 months ahead) and predicting response to treatment, but early treatment based on the tumour marker alone does not give a survival advantage. Approximately 60% of patients with ovarian cancer will relapse at some point. Hormonal approaches using tamoxifen or aromatase inhibitors can slow down the rate of progression and delay onset of symptoms.

Complications

Advanced disease will spread in a transcoelomic manner, producing ascites, and can produce subacute or complete bowel obstruction due to serosal involvement of the bowel. A pelvic mass can result in hydronephrosis due to ureteric obstruction. Ascites may require frequent paracentesis, and talc pleurodesis can reduce the recurrence of pleural effusions. Patients with ovarian cancer are at a particularly high risk of thrombosis (DVT, PE) due to a prothrombotic tendency that correlates with the disease activity. Furthermore, thrombosis can occur despite adequate anticoagulation.

Prognosis

Prognosis correlates with stage at diagnosis. Overall 5-year survival is 30% but ranges from >90% for stage 1 to <25% for stage 4. Patients who have disease resistant to platinum therapy, large volume residual disease following debulking, or clear cell histology all have a worse outcome. Patients with BRCA gene mutations are more likely to have visceral metastasis, but equally are more likely to respond to platinum therapy and have longer treatment-free intervals. The best predictor of outcome is for patients who achieve complete cytoreduction at initial surgery.

Figure 38.1 Clinical features of endometrial cancer

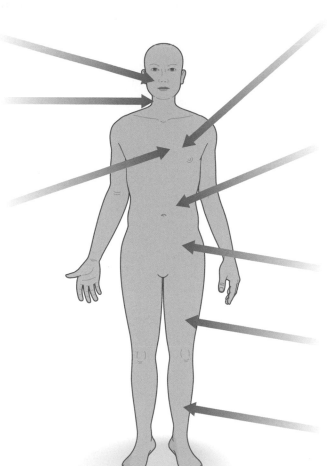

Face
- Conjunctival pallor
- Icterus, jaundice

Lymph nodes
- Neck
- Supraclavicular
- Axillary
- Inguinal
- Para-aortic

Cardiovascular
- Pericardial effusion
- Loud P2 (pulmonary hypertension, PE)

Observation
- Ascites
- Cachexia (advanced disease)
- Dehydration (due to nausea)
- Nausea and vomiting
- PV discharge
- PV bleeding
- Dyspareunia
- Haematuria

Other
- PR examination
- PV examination

Respiratory
- Pleural effusion
- Pleural rub (PE)
- Tachypnoea (PE)

Abdomen
- Surgical scars
- Visible peristalsis
- Bowel obstruction
- Abdominal distension
- Ascites
- Hepatomegaly
- Hepatic tenderness
- Renal tenderness (hydroureter)
- Pelvic mass
- Adenexal mass

Neurological
- Focal neurological signs (brain metastasis)

Skeletal survey
- Focal bone tenderness (metastases) (pelvis, spine, long bones)

Periphery
- Calf tenderness (DVT)

Table 38.1 Risk factors for endometrial cancer

	High oestrogen levels	Low progestogen levels
Endogenous	• Obesity • Ovarian granulosa cell tumour	• Polycystic ovarian syndrome • Nulliparity • Early menarche • Late menopause
Exogenous	• Oestrogen-only HRT • Tamoxifen	

Table 38.2 FIGO staging of endometrial cancer

Stage	Definition
1a	Disease in the body of uterus, invasion <50% myometrium
1b	Disease in the body of the uterus, invasion >50% myometrium
2	Disease in the body of the uterus and cervix
3a	Disease advanced within the pelvis, involvement of the ovaries
3b	Disease advanced within the pelvis, involvement of the vagina and parametrium
3c	Disease advanced within the pelvis, involvement of the local lymph nodes
4a	Disease spread to outside the pelvis, involvement of the bowel or bladder
4b	Disease spread to outside the pelvis, involvement of more distant organs

Epidemiology

Endometrial cancer is the fifth most common cancer in women in the UK. It largely affects post-menopausal women, particularly those aged 60–79 years and accounts for 5% of all female cancers.

It is the most common type of cancer of the uterus and the majority of cases are adenocarcinoma, of which there are three types: endometrioid (commonest), papillary serous and clear cell (rare). Carcinosarcoma of the uterus is rare and behaves in a more aggressive manner.

Aetiology

A high level of oestrogen unopposed by progestogen is associated with an increased risk of endometrial cancer. Therefore, factors that result in excess oestrogen levels or low progestogen levels increase a woman's risk of endometrial cancer (Table 38.1).

Other factors associated with an increased risk of endometrial cancer include hypertension, diabetes mellitus, Lynch type II syndrome and endometrial hyperplasia with atypia (benign).

Protective factors include history of pregnancy and combined oral contraceptive pill use.

Clinical presentation

Endometrial cancer tends to present early, with post-menopausal bleeding (PMB), intermenstrual bleeding or recent-onset menorrhagia. All women over the age of 45 years presenting with PMB should be investigated. Other less common symptoms include lower abdominal discomfort, vaginal discharge and dyspareunia. On bimanual palpation and speculum examination the pelvis often appears normal.

Advanced disease may cause urinary frequency, fatigue, loss of appetite, back pain and constipation. Spread of endometrial cancer usually occurs directly through the myometrium to the cervix and vagina. Metastases occur via the lymphatic system but haematogenous spread occurs late and therefore widespread metastasis at presentation is unusual.

Investigations and staging

A transvaginal ultrasound scan is performed to assess endometrial thickness. In post-menopausal women, an endometrial thickness >4 mm is suggestive but not diagnostic of endometrial cancer. Endometrial thickness is not a reliable indicator in premenopausal women because endometrial thickness varies during the menstrual cycle.

An endometrial biopsy is required to confirm the diagnosis. It can be obtained using a pipelle, hysteroscopy or dilatation and curettage. A pipelle cannot diagnose cancer because it does not assess if the basement membrane is breached.

A blood sample may be taken to measure the tumour marker CA125. This is neither sensitive nor specific for endometrial cancer but can be useful for disease monitoring.

If investigations confirm endometrial cancer, a chest X-ray is performed to check for pulmonary metastases, and investigation by CT is required. A pelvic MRI scan can assess the size and extent of invasion of the tumour into the cervix and myometrium.

If indicated, an examination under anaesthesia may be performed to assess the size and mobility of the uterus and any involvement of the vagina, cervix, bladder, or rectum. Advanced disease can cause hydronephrosis and patients can present with renal impairment.

Endometrial cancer is staged using the FIGO staging system, which is based on surgical and histological findings. Hence accurate staging requires an operative procedure (Table 38.2).

Treatment

Treatment depends on the stage and grade of the cancer and the general health of the woman.

For patients with stage 1a cancers, surgery with total abdominal hysterectomy and bilateral salpingo-oopherectomy is usually sufficient treatment. When the tumour is confined to the inner third of the myometrium, the likelihood of lymph node involvement is low. The majority of women with endometrial cancer will have early stage disease.

In women with stage 1b or 2 disease, or for high-grade cancers, adjuvant pelvic radiotherapy is given, which reduces the rate of local recurrence.

Radiotherapy may be used as the primary treatment in women unfit to undergo surgery or in women with locally advanced disease (stage 3 and 4a).

For patients with recurrent disease, hormonal therapy using progestogens can be used to slow the growth of the cancer. The best response rates to endocrine therapy correlate with well-differentiated histology, a long disease-free interval following primary treatment and increased expression of progesterone receptors. The response rate to progesterone therapy is 25% with a progression-free survival of 4 months.

Chemotherapy using carboplatin and paclitaxel, or cisplatin and doxorubicin can improve disease control and symptoms in patients with recurrent disease but the impact on survival is limited. There is limited benefit for chemotherapy given in an adjuvant setting and no advantage to combining hormonal and chemotherapy.

Complications

Patients who receive pelvic radiotherapy are at risk of short-term side effects including diarrhoea, cystitis, nausea and tiredness. Longer-term effects include early menopause, vaginal dryness, urinary frequency due to bladder wall fibrosis and persistent diarrhoea. Progestogen therapy is associated with water retention, breast tenderness, nausea and tiredness.

Prognosis

Endometrial cancer has the best prognosis of all the gynaecological cancers. Poor prognostic indicators include older age, advanced stage, high-grade tumours and adenosquamous histology. Recurrent disease is most common at the vaginal vault and often presents within 2–3 years of the primary treatment.

Stage	5-year overall survival (%)
1	80
2	70–80
3	40–50
4	20–30

Figure 39.1 Clinical features of cervical cancer

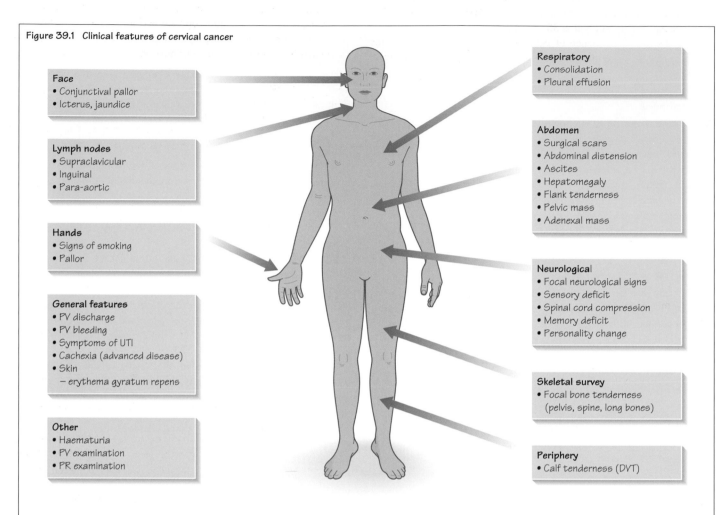

Face
• Conjunctival pallor
• Icterus, jaundice

Lymph nodes
• Supraclavicular
• Inguinal
• Para-aortic

Hands
• Signs of smoking
• Pallor

General features
• PV discharge
• PV bleeding
• Symptoms of UTI
• Cachexia (advanced disease)
• Skin
    – erythema gyratum repens

Other
• Haematuria
• PV examination
• PR examination

Respiratory
• Consolidation
• Pleural effusion

Abdomen
• Surgical scars
• Abdominal distension
• Ascites
• Hepatomegaly
• Flank tenderness
• Pelvic mass
• Adenexal mass

Neurological
• Focal neurological signs
• Sensory deficit
• Spinal cord compression
• Memory deficit
• Personality change

Skeletal survey
• Focal bone tenderness
    (pelvis, spine, long bones)

Periphery
• Calf tenderness (DVT)

Table 39.1 FIGO staging of cervical cancer

Stage	Definition
0	Pre-invasive disease, CIN 1–3
1a1	Stromal invasion only with a maximum depth of 3mm and no wider than 7mm
1a2	Stromal invasion only with a depth >3mm but <5mm and no wider than 7mm
1b1	Clinical lesion confined to cervix greater than stage 1a and less than 4cm in size
1b2	Clinical lesion confined to cervix but greater than 4cm in size
2a	Tumour extends beyond cervix, no obvious parametrial involvement. Involvement of up to the upper two-thirds of vagina
2b	Obvious parametrial involvement but not into the pelvic side wall
3a	Tumour not extending into the pelvic side wall but involves lower third of vagina
3b	Extension into the pelvic side wall, or hydronephrosis, or non-functioning kidney
4a	Tumour spread to involve adjacent organs outside of the true pelvis
4b	Distant metastasis

Epidemiology

In the UK, cervical cancer is the seventh most common female cancer, representing 2.5% of all cancer cases. Worldwide it represents 10% of all female cancers and 80% occur in the developing world. The average age at presentation is 35–44 years.

The decline in incidence of cervical cancer has been due to the introduction of screening programmes based on cytological cervical smear assessment.

Aetiology

Invasive cervical cancer most commonly, progresses from cervical infection by human papilloma virus (HPV) to cervical intraepithelial neoplasia (CIN) and on to invasive disease. CIN is a cytological diagnosis and describes the involvement of the epidermis:
- CIN 1: involvement of lower 1/3 of epithelium;
- CIN 2: involvement of lower 2/3 of epithelium;
- CIN 3: involvement of all layers of epithelium.

Cervical cancer develops when disease breaches the epithelial basement membrane and invades the cervical stroma. The majority of cervical cancers are squamous cell, but adenocarcinoma accounts for 15% of cases. Adenocarcinoma develops from the endocervical epithelium and most commonly affects women under 40 years of age.

The most significant causative factor is HPV, particularly HPV 16, 18, 31, 33 and 45. HPV 16 and 18 convey the highest risk of malignancy. Other risk factors include high number of sexual partners, early age at first intercourse, low socioeconomic status, non-barrier forms of contraception, cigarette smoking, prolonged use of combined oral contraceptive pill, multiparity and immunocompromised state (e.g. HIV).

Vaccination against HPV is now available in the form of Cervarix, which protects against HPV 16 and 18, and Gardasil which protects against HPV 6, 11, 16 and 18, thus it prevents many cases of genital warts as well as cervical cancer. Cervarix is now offered to 12- to 13-year-old girls in the UK.

Clinical presentation

CIN and microinvasive disease are asymptomatic. Early stage invasive disease presents with post-coital bleeding, intermenstrual bleeding, postmenopausal bleeding or offensive vaginal discharge. Pain is not commonly associated with early stage disease, but symptoms might be suggestive of a urinary tract infection.

In the later stages of the disease, involvement of the ureters, bladder, rectum and nerves leads to uraemia, haematuria, rectal bleeding, back pain, referred pain in the legs and deep lateral pain. Mass effect of a bulky tumour may result in increased urinary frequency and altered bowel habit.

On bimanual palpation and speculum examination the cervix often appears normal in CIN and microinvasive disease. A palpable cervical mass may only be apparent in invasive disease.

Investigations and staging

Colposcopy is performed to visualise the cervix. Acetic acid is applied to the cervix and the presence of leukoplakia (white epithelium), mosaic structure and punctation on the cervix are features of pre-invasive disease. Abnormal vascularity is suggestive of invasive disease. A punch or loop biopsy is obtained during colposcopy for histological examination and allows confirmation of diagnosis. Symptomatic patients require examination under anaesthetic to establish the extent of disease. Cervical cancer is staged using the FIGO system, where the divisions are histological and does not include lymph node involvement (Table 39.1). The majority of cases are stage 1 or 2.

Cystoscopy and sigmoidoscopy are performed if there is suspicion of adjacent organ involvement. A CT or MRI scan of the pelvis and abdomen is used to assess tumour bulk and lymphadenopathy.

Screening

The national cervical screening programme offers a cervical smear every 3 years to women aged 25–49 years and every 5 years to women aged 50–64 years. Cervical smears use cytology to detect abnormal cells and prompt intervention can prevent invasive cancer developing.

Screening following treatment

Patients are reviewed with cervical smears and clinical examination.
CIN 1: repeat at 6 months, 12 months and then yearly for a further 2 years.
CIN 2, 3: repeat at 6 months, 12 months and then yearly for a further 8 years.
Invasive disease: repeat at 3 months, 6 months and then every 6 months for 5 years.

Treatment

Optimum treatment is determined by the stage of the disease, age and general health of the woman, and plans for future fertility.
- Local excision using loop diathermy is performed for CIN 2/3 confined to the visible ectocervix.
- Loop biopsy is performed for CIN 3 with disease extending into cervical canal.
- Simple hysterectomy is performed for microinvasive disease.
- Stage 1b or 2 cervical cancers are treated by radical hysterectomy with pelvic lymphadenectomy or pelvic radiotherapy. Both methods are equally effective.
- Stage 2b and 3 should be treated with pelvic radiotherapy, and patients treated with curative intent typically receive chemoradiotherapy with cisplatin as a radiation sensitiser.
- Stage 4 and recurrent disease are treated with chemotherapy. Radiotherapy can be used to treat specific site of metastasis.

Chemotherapy alone has no role in the adjuvant treatment of cervical cancer.

Prognosis

Poor prognosis is associated with adenocarcinoma, lymph node involvement, advanced clinical stage, large primary tumour and early recurrence. Relapse after 5 years is unusual.

Stage of cervical cancer	5-year overall survival (%)
1a	100
1b	70–90
2	50–70
3	25–60
4	10–20

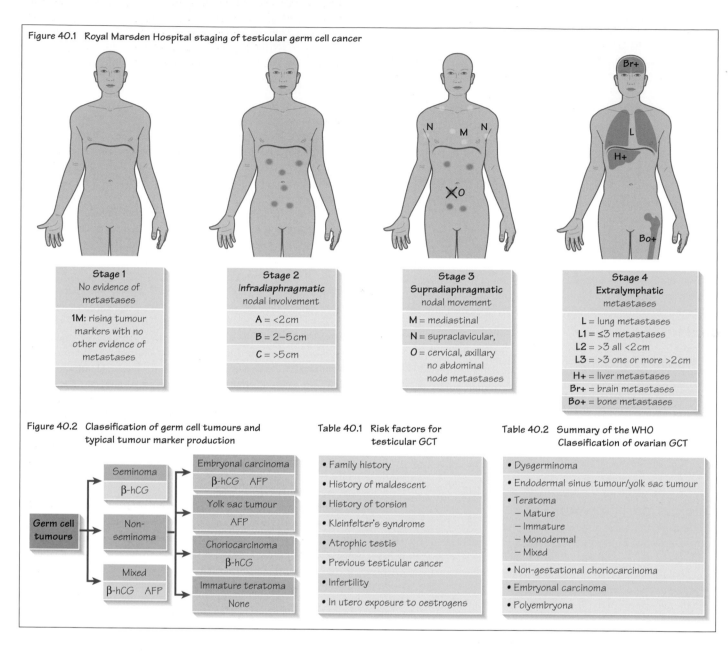

Figure 40.1 Royal Marsden Hospital staging of testicular germ cell cancer

Stage 1
No evidence of metastases

1M: rising tumour markers with no other evidence of metastases

Stage 2
Infradiaphragmatic nodal involvement

A = <2cm
B = 2–5cm
C = >5cm

Stage 3
Supradiaphragmatic nodal movement

M = mediastinal
N = supraclavicular,
O = cervical, axillary no abdominal node metastases

Stage 4
Extralymphatic metastases

L = lung metastases
L1 = ≤3 metastases
L2 = >3 all <2cm
L3 = >3 one or more >2cm
H+ = liver metastases
Br+ = brain metastases
Bo+ = bone metastases

Figure 40.2 Classification of germ cell tumours and typical tumour marker production

Germ cell tumours
- Seminoma — β-hCG
- Non-seminoma
- Mixed — β-hCG AFP

- Embryonal carcinoma — β-hCG AFP
- Yolk sac tumour — AFP
- Choriocarcinoma — β-hCG
- Immature teratoma — None

Table 40.1 Risk factors for testicular GCT

- Family history
- History of maldescent
- History of torsion
- Kleinfelter's syndrome
- Atrophic testis
- Previous testicular cancer
- Infertility
- In utero exposure to oestrogens

Table 40.2 Summary of the WHO Classification of ovarian GCT

- Dysgerminoma
- Endodermal sinus tumour/yolk sac tumour
- Teratoma
  - Mature
  - Immature
  - Monodermal
  - Mixed
- Non-gestational choriocarcinoma
- Embryonal carcinoma
- Polyembryona

Epidemiology

Germ cell tumours (GCT) are rare, but account for 95% of testicular tumours and 3–5% of ovarian malignancies. They are the commonest cancer in men aged 20–40 years and the peak incidence of ovarian GCT is in young women and adolescent girls. They represent one of the few groups of solid tumours for which the majority of patients can expect to be cured.

Extra-gonadal tumours account for less than 10% of all germ cell tumours. They occur in midline structures, most commonly in the mediastinum (50–70%) and retroperitoneum (30–40%), and rarely the brain, head and neck. In the mediastinum the peak incidence is in the third decade of life.

Aetiology

A family history of testicular cancer is one of the strongest risk factors for disease, although a definite genetic link has not yet been identified. More than 80% of testicular cancers express 12p gain, often as an isochromosome of 12p (i12p), where one arm of the chromosome is lost and replaced with an exact replica of the other arm.

Carcinoma in situ (intratubular neoplasia) is the precursor of testicular germ cell cancer and is found in addition to the invasive component.

Pathophysiology
Seminoma and dysgerminoma
Seminoma accounts for 50% of malignant germ cell tumours in men, with a peak incidence between the ages of 30 and 40. Spermatic seminoma is more common in older men, between the ages of 60 and 70. Ovarian dysgerminoma is directly comparable with testicular seminoma and accounts for the majority of cases of ovarian GCT.

The majority of patients (75%) present with disease confined to the testis or ovary. Spread is usually predictable from para-aortic to supradiaphragmatic nodes, and then to extranodal sites. Growth is slow, and microscopic disease may take up to 10 years to present clinically. Seminomas and dysgerminomas do not produce a reliable tumour marker with which to monitor disease, but hCG can be elevated in 10–25% of cases.

Non-seminoma
Disease spread occurs earlier than in seminomas, and therefore only 50% of patients present with localised disease. AFP and hCG tumour markers are elevated in approximately 75% of cases.

Clinical presentation
Testicular tumours present as a painless solid mass in the scrotum, with enlargement of the testicle, scrotal pain, back pain, a dragging sensation in the scrotum, or gynaecomastia (due to high circulating hCG levels). Features may be similar to epididymo-orchitis, but should raise suspicion if they persist after a course of antibiotics.

Ovarian GCTs grow rapidly and the duration of symptoms before presentation is usually 2–4 weeks. There is commonly abdominal pain and a palpable abdominal or pelvic mass causing abdominal distension. Ascites or peritonitis may occur secondary to torsion, infection, or rupture. Vaginal bleeding is relatively uncommon. There may be bowel or urinary obstruction, particularly with large masses.

Metastatic disease can manifest as dyspnoea, cough, SVC obstruction, CNS symptoms and liver capsular pain.

Extragonadal tumours may present with chest pain, dyspnoea, SVC obstruction, dysphagia, hoarseness and cough. In the retro-peritoneum, patients experience few symptoms until the tumour is advanced, as it expands without acutely obstructing vital organs. Patients may present with an abdominal mass and abdominal or back pain. Intracranial tumours are extremely rare and present with features of raised intracranial pressure. In more severe cases, neurological symptoms may be overt and be associated with endocrine dysfunction.

Investigations and staging
Serum tumour markers; alpha-fetoprotein (AFP), β-human chorionic gonadotrophin (hCG) and lactate dehydrogenase (LDH) are expressed in varying patterns depending on tumour type. LDH is a good prognostic indicator as it correlates to tumour bulk.

Staging is based on tumour markers and CT scan findings (Figure 40.2). The International Germ Cell Consensus Classification uses these factors to determine disease prognosis.

Ovarian GCT should be suspected in all young women presenting with a pelvic mass, and requires measurement of AFP, hCG and LDH. Elevation of CA125 is unusual. CT imaging of chest, abdomen and pelvis is required.

Extragonadal tumours may produce placental alkaline phosphatase, and gonadal examination and ultrasound for a hidden primary is required, as this alters treatment options and outcomes. CT imaging of the chest, abdomen, thorax (and head if relevant) should be arranged. Genetic analysis may be relevant as trisomy 8 is associated with 16% of cases, as is Kleinfelter syndrome in 14–20%. The tumour should be biopsied and the histological features are the same as for gonadal tumours.

Treatment
For **testicular GCT**, the management of stage 1 disease is radical inguinal orchidectomy, with clamping of the spermatic cord at the internal inguinal ring to prevent tumour seeding. Postoperative tumour markers are monitored during surveillance and if the decline is slow, residual disease is possible. The relapse rate after surgery is 20% for seminoma and 30% for non-seminoma tumours. In seminoma, adjuvant radiotherapy to the para-aortic lymph nodes or one cycle of carboplatin can reduce the risk of relapse. In non-seminoma GCT, two cycles of BEP chemotherapy can reduce relapse.

In stages 2a and 2b seminoma, radiotherapy to the para-aortic and iliac lymph nodes is indicated. For all other stages of all forms of GCT, orchidectomy is delayed, as chemotherapy is the mainstay of treatment. In good prognosis disease, three cycles of bleomycin, etopiside and cisplatin (BEP) chemotherapy are used, with weekly monitoring of tumour markers, and post-treatment CT imaging for response assessment. Orchidectomy is performed after chemotherapy.

Ovarian GCTs are treated with optimal cytoreductive surgery with preservation of fertility considered wherever possible. Total abdominal hysterectomy with bilateral salpingo-ophorectomy is therefore avoided in favour of unilateral salpingo-oophorectomy, omentectomy, peritoneal washings and detailed inspection of the abdominal cavity. Biopsies of common sites of spread are taken for staging. Pelvic and para-aortic lymph nodes are biopsied if suspicious. Biopsy of the contralateral ovary is not routine, unless macroscopically abnormal, as potential adhesions or ovarian failure can affect fertility. If it is abnormal, biopsy or ovarian cystectomy is performed, followed by BSO if a frozen section demonstrates malignancy or gonadal dysgenesis. Dysgerminoma is the exception, as 10–15% may have bilateral involvement. Patients receive post-operative chemotherapy with three cycles of BEP, unless there is bulky residual disease, in which case four cycles are given.

Extragonadal GCTs are treated dependent on the site and histological type of tumour. Seminomas are chemotherapy and radiotherapy sensitive, whereas non-seminomas are less so and chemotherapy is given post surgery. For mediastinal and retroperitoneal tumours BEP chemotherapy and surgery are treatments of choice. In intracranial tumours, radiotherapy is given alone in seminoma and in combination with chemotherapy in non-seminoma. Surgery may remove residual mass after chemotherapy, but carries a risk of spinal metastases.

Prognosis
Patients with non-seminoma, good prognosis disease have a 5-year survival of 92–95%, intermediate prognosis tumours have a 70–80% and 48% 5-year survival for poor-prognosis patients. Patients with pure seminoma are described as having a good or intermediate prognosis.

Figure 41.1 Clinical features of prostate cancer

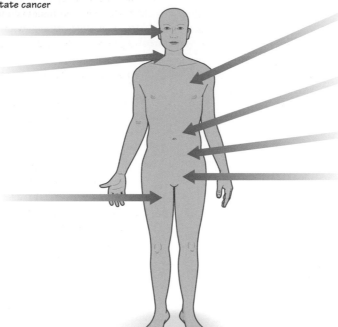

Face
- Conjunctival pallor
- Icterus, jaundice

Lymph nodes
- Inguinal
- Para-aortic
- Supraclavicular
- Axillary

Symptoms
- Bone pain
- Urinary dribbling
- Poor urine flow

Skeletal survey
- Focal bone tenderness
- Pathological fracture
  (pelvis, spine, long bones)

Observation
- Ascites
- Cachexia
- Dehydration
- Fatigue
- Anorexia

Respiratory
- Tachypnoea
- Stridor
- Consolidation
- Pleural effusion

Abdomen
- Abdominal distension
- Ascites
- Hepatomegaly

Neurological
- Confusion
- Focal neurological signs

Spinal cord compression
- Bowel dysfunction
- Faecal incontinence
- Constipation
- Bladder dysfunction
- Retention
- Dribbling
- Incontinence
- Back pain
- Localised to site of collapse
- Radicular
  – may move down limbs
  – unresolving pain
  – worse with cough or straining
  – limb weakness

Table 41.1 TNM staging of prostate cancer

Classification	Division	Description
T – extent of tumour	T0	No tumour palpable
	T1	Tumour in one lobe of the prostate
	T2	Tumour involving both prostate lobes
	T3	Tumour infiltrating out of the prostate to involve seminal vesicles
	T4	Extensive tumour, fixed and infiltrating local structures
N – regional lymph nodes	N0	No lymph node involvement
	N1	Ispilateral lymph nodes involved
	N2	Bilateral lymph node involved
	N3	Fixed regional lymph nodes
	N4	Juxtaregional lymph nodes
M – metastasis	M0	No metastasis
	M1	Distant metastasis

Table 41.2
Prognosis of prostate cancer

Type of tumour	5-year overall survival (%)
Incidental	85
Early localised	78
Locally advanced	60
Metastatic	10–30
Overall	65

Epidemiology

Prostate cancer is the most common cancer in men in the UK, with approximately 32 000 new cases per year and 10 000 deaths. More than 60% of cases occur in men over 70 years of age. Nearly 50% have metastatic disease at presentation and in a further 25% the disease presents with localised extracapsular spread. It has been estimated that for a 50-year-old man, the projected lifetime risk of histological evidence of prostate cancer is 42%, risk of clinical disease is 9.5% and risk of death from prostate cancer is 3%.

The incidence of prostate cancer increases with age; only 12% of clinically apparent cases arise before the age of 65 and only 20% of deaths occur in men under 70 years old.

Substantial increases in incidence have been reported in recent years in many countries around the world, after correction for an ageing population. Some of this may be due to a real increase in risk, but additionally the increased use of transurethral resection of the prostate (TURP) and PSA testing have increased the detection rate. In the USA, the reported incidence is up to 10 times higher than in

UK, most likely due to the effect of widespread prostate cancer screening.

Aetiology and pathophysiology

Prostate cancers are mostly adenocarcinomas, with 70% occurring in the peripheral zone, 20% in the transitional zone and 10% in the central zone. Family history is a feature in 10% of cases and such patients may develop prostate cancer at a younger age. Inherited *BRCA1* and *BRCA2* mutations (breast–ovarian cancer families) and hereditary prostate cancers due to mutations of *HPC1* (chromosome 1q24–q25) and *HPC2* (chromosome Xq27–q28) have been implicated in hereditary prostate cancer (see Chapter 8). There are racial differences in the incidence of prostate cancer; the order of frequency is Black > Caucasian > Oriental. The role of diet remains controversial, although high-fat, low-fibre, smoked foods and dairy produce may increase the risk, while soya beans and retinoids appear to be protective against prostate cancer. The incidence of prostate cancer in vegetarians is 50–75% that of omnivores.

Clinical presentation

Men with prostate cancer confined to the prostate often are completely asymptomatic. Those with a large component of benign prostatic hyperplasia but transitional zone disease, often present with bladder outlet obstruction but have no other signs of prostate cancer and are diagnosed via transurethral resection.

The most frequent presentation of locally advanced disease is with urinary frequency, a poor urine flow or difficulty starting or stopping urination. Associated features include bone pain from metastatic disease, lethargy, and rarely weight loss and bilateral leg oedema.

Patients can be referred following screen detection of a raised prostate-specific antigen (PSA), accounting for 2–6% of UK cases.

Investigations and staging

Patients require a careful history and full clinical examination, including rectal examination and survey for focal bone tenderness. Routine blood tests required are serum PSA, full blood count, acid phosphatase, alkaline phosphatase and serum biochemistry. PSA is a serine protease that dissolves prostatic coagulum and can be raised in benign prostatic hypertrophy. With PSA levels between 4 and 10 µg/L, the likelihood of the patient having prostate cancer is 25%, above these levels the likelihood increases to 40%.

Plain X-rays of the chest and any sites of bone pain should be performed. Patients require a transrectal ultrasound and bone scan.

The staging classification is outlined in Table 41.1. The tumour grade can be well, moderately or poorly differentiated and is elaborated in the Gleason grade, which scores the tumours on a scale of 1–10, where 10 is the most poorly differentiated. Transurethral ultrasound has a low specificity for malignancy but a high specificity for assessing the integrity of the prostatic capsule. It is often combined with a needle biopsy where at least six cores of tissue are sampled. MR or CT imaging is used to investigate lymph node involvement.

Treatment

Early-stage disease (T1, T2) can be treated with 'watchful waiting', radiotherapy, or radical prostatectomy. There is no evidence to support the superiority of any of these approaches. Watchful waiting varies from waiting until the patient presents with symptoms, to more active follow-up of outpatients with regular PSA testing and physical examination. Although this strategy does not produce the physical or sexual complications associated with other treatments, it may increase anxiety. It is the best option for men with low-grade, incidentally detected tumours and those who have a life expectancy of <10 years. For patients with a longer life expectancy, treatment will improve the local control rate but may adversely affect their quality of life.

Radical radiotherapy is the most common treatment used in the UK. Complications include damage to adjacent organs causing acute diarrhoea (50%), chronic proctitis (5–10%), incontinence (about 1–6%) and impotence (40%). The complications of radical prostatectomy include operative mortality (0.5%), complete incontinence (1–27%) and impotence (20–85%). The published survival data for radiotherapy are worse than for surgery, but less fit patients will be referred for radiotherapy rather than surgery. For younger patients with poor histology, surgery has a better outcome than radiotherapy.

Locally advanced disease (T3, T4) or **metastatic disease** is treated by endocrine therapy with orchidectomy, LHRH antagonists with or without antiandrogens (such as flutamide, bicalutamide and cyproterone acetate), or oestrogens. Orchidectomy is associated with major psychological side effects, impotence and hot flushes. LHRH antagonists cause an initial increase in testosterone levels that can cause tumour flare for the first 1–2 weeks. This may result in disease progression causing spinal cord compression, ureteric obstruction, or increasing bone pain. For this reason, an antiandrogen should be started 3–7 days before the LHRH analogue injection and be continued for 3 weeks after it. The advantage of using a combination of LHRH analogues and antiandrogens to maximally suppress androgen levels has been demonstrated in some studies, and a meta-analysis of all the trials showed a modest survival benefit over LHRH agonist alone.

Metastatic bone pain may be relieved by irradiation to localised sites or, if extensive, hemibody single fraction radiotherapy. An alternative is intravenous strontium (^{89}Sr) isotope, which is taken up avidly by bone.

New approaches using chemotherapy are under evaluation but most chemotherapeutic approaches have produced disappointing results with response rates typically <20%. Agents such as docetaxel, cabazitaxel and abiraterone provide palliation in advanced disease, and anti-angiogenic agents such as thalidomide are under study.

Screening

See Chapter 16 for a discussion on prostate cancer screening.

Prognosis

Despite the effectiveness of initial hormonal therapy, metastatic prostate cancer is an incurable disease, with patients surviving a median of 6–9 months after the development of androgen insensitivity. In patients with small bulk localised disease and well- to moderately differentiated tumours, the survival is 80% at 10 years.

Patients with poorly differentiated tumours and high Gleason grade have a worse prognosis with observation and radiotherapy (15% 10-year survival) than with surgery (60–80% 10-year survival). It is possible that there is selection bias as only those who are fit will be referred for surgery, with those unfit referred for radiotherapy.

Table 42.1 TNM staging of bladder cancer

Classification	Division	Description
T – extent of tumour	Tis	Carcinoma in situ (malignant cells not invading the basement membrane)
	Ta	Non-invasive papillary carcinoma
	T1	Superficial tumour, not invading beyond the lamina propria
	T2a	Tumour invading into the inner half of the muscle layer
	T2b	Tumour invading into the outer half of the muscle layer
	T3a	Microscopic tumour involving the serosal surface of the bladder
	T3b	Macroscopic tumour involving the serosal surface of the bladder
	T4a	Tumour spread to the stroma of the prostate (in men), or to the uterus and/or vagina (in women)
	T4b	Tumour spread to the pelvic wall or the abdominal wall
N – regional lymph nodes	N0	No lymph node involvement
	N1	One affected lymph node in the true pelvis
	N2	Two or more affected lymph nodes in the true pelvis
	N3	Involved lymph nodes along the common iliac artery
M – metastasis	M0	No metastases
	M1	Distant metastases

Table 42.2 Robson's staging of renal cancer

Classification	Division	Description
T – extent of tumour	T0	No evidence of primary tumour
	T1	<7cm and limited to kidney
	T2	>7cm limited to kidney
	T3	Tumour extension to major veins or adrenal glands or perinephric tissue but not beyond Gerota's fascia
	T3a	Tumour invades adrenal gland or perinephric tissue
	T3b	Tumour invasion to renal veins and inferior vena cava below diaphragm
	T3c	Tumour invasion into inferior vena cava above the diaphragm
	T4	Tumour invasion beyond Gerota's fascia and involvement more than one regional lymph node
N – regional lymph nodes	N0	No regional lymph node metastases
	N1	Metastases in single regional lymph node
	N2	Metastases in more than one regional lymph node
M – metastasis	M0	No distant metastasis
	M1	Distant metastasis

Epidemiology

Bladder cancer accounts for 5% of cancer registrations in the UK for men and 2% for women, with 10 000 new cases per year. There is a ratio of male:female ratio of 3:1 and peak incidence around 65 years of age. It is the fourth most common cancer in men.

Adult renal cancer accounts for 3% of adult malignancies in men and 1% in women and most are in patients over 50 years of age.

Aetiology

Worldwide, chronic bladder infection from parasites such as schistosomiosis is the most common risk factor for bladder cancer. In the Western world risk factors include environmental exposure to inflammation from smoking, arylamines (in the dye industry) and rubber processing. Mutations on chromosome 9, particularly the *TP53* gene have an increased risk of transitional cell cancer (TCC). Overexpression of EGFR is reported in 40% of cases and correlates with poor prognosis.

Adult renal cell cancer is more common in men and those who smoke. It can be seen in Von Hippel–Lindau disease (an autosomal dominant condition with mutations on chromosome 3) and familial papillary renal carcinoma syndrome (due to a mutation of *MET* oncogene on chromosome 7q31) (see Chapter 8). Renal metastasis can arise from lung or breast cancers, melanoma, or lymphoma.

Pathophysiology

Transitional cells are stem cells adjacent to the basement membrane of the epithelial surface that line the renal tract, from the renal papillae to the proximal urethra. Squamous epithelium lines the distal urethra. Most transitional cell tumours arise in the bladder, as this is an area of polyclonal field change most susceptible to malignant change. Many cancers start as papillary tumours, which can be multifocal over the surface area of the bladder. At diagnosis, 70% of patients will have superficial papillary disease and 30% invasive tumour, 10% of TCC start as carcinoma in situ (CIS) as flat, non-invasive, high-grade bladder cancers that spread over the surface of the bladder. They then become invasive and penetrate the bladder muscle before they metastasise. Up to 95% of bladder tumours are transitional cell carcinoma and 5% are squamous cell carcinomas, usually as a result of chronic inflammation. Other rare tumour types include rhabdomyosarcoma and leiomyosarcoma.

More than 90% of renal tumours arise in the cortex, probably from cells of the proximal convoluted tubule. They are named renal cell carcinoma, renal adenocarcinoma, clear cell carcinoma, or hypernephroma, which are synonymous. The remaining 10% arise from the renal pelvis and are transitional cell carcinomas that resemble tumours of the ureter, bladder and urethra. The tumour cells can produce excess hormones such as erythropoietin, rennin, or PTH-related polypeptide (PTHrP), causing polycythaemia, hypertension, or hypercalcaemia respectively.

Clinical presentation

The majority of patients with bladder cancer (80–90%) present with painless haematuria. A bladder mass or obstructed kidney can be palpable and distant metastases are uncommon (5%). Some patients can have symptoms of infection, such as urgency and dysuria, and sterile pyuria can occur. Systemic effects are uncommon.

Renal cancer can present with haematuria but is more commonly associated with loin, back, or abdominal pain. Spread can be local via the lymphatics to the renal hilum, retroperitoneum, or para-aortic lymph nodes. Varicocoeles can be a feature in male patients with occlusion of the right or left testicular veins, which drain respectively into the left renal vein and IVC. Metastases from renal cell cancer typically present in the lung, liver, bones and brain, and systemic effects can manifest with fever, weight loss, gynaecomastia, night sweats, Cushing's syndrome, polymyositis, dermatomyositis, malaise and anaemia. Increasing numbers of renal tumours are diagnosed as incidental findings following abdominal imaging for other reasons.

Investigations and staging

All patients who present with painless haematuria should have urinalysis, urine cytology and be considered for cystoscopy with evaluation of the bladder mucosa and urethra. Patients with positive cytology but normal cystoscopy should have examination of the upper tracts and for male patients, a prostate examination. Definitive diagnosis can be established only by cystoscopy and biopsy.

CT imaging of the abdomen and pelvis can detect local extension and lymph node involvement. Imaging of the chest can screen for pulmonary metastasis. Bone scan is recommended for any patient with bone pain or raised alkaline phosphatase.

Blood tests should include renal and liver function, PT, PTT and calcium. There are no specific tumour markers. Staging classification is outlined in Tables 42.1 and 42.2.

Treatment

Bladder cancer

Superficial bladder cancer is treated by transurethral resection (TURBT). Features that increase the risk of relapse include high-grade histology, incomplete resection, multifocal disease and carcinoma in situ. Such patients should be considered for adjuvant intravesical Bacillus Calmette–Guérin (BCG) therapy. Muscle invasive bladder cancer options range from TURBT to radical cystectomy or radical radiotherapy, depending on the age and performance status of the patient. Recent advances in radiotherapy from improved CT simulation have meant more accurate treatment, with improved outcome results and reduced side effects.

Metastatic disease may be treated with combination chemotherapy using gemcitabine and cisplatin in patients with good functional status, although complete remissions are rare.

Renal cancer

Where possible, radical nephrectomy should be undertaken as it may be curative for early stage disease. Surgery can palliate symptoms of haematuria and pain in patients with locally advanced disease, and improve duration of survival in patients with metastatic disease subsequently treated with immunotherapy. Spontaneous regression of metastases following nephrectomy, although well recognised, is extremely rare. Adjuvant therapy does not improve survival.

Standard chemotherapy has little effect in renal cancer. Biological therapies with antiangiogenesis inhibitors such as everolimus, temsirolimus, sorafenib, sunitinib and axitinib can produce improvements in disease control and survival. Immunotherapy with interferon or interleukin-2 may be used in the management of metastatic disease and can induce complete remissions or durable partial remissions in approximately 10–15% of patients.

Prognosis

The prognosis of patients with bladder cancer correlates with the degree of invasion at diagnosis. Other prognostic determinants include age, performance status, gender, histological grade of tumour, and size and extent of tumour spread. The 5-year survival for superficial cancers is 80–90% and for invasive cancer is 30–40%.

The 5-year survival for renal cell cancer is 45%.

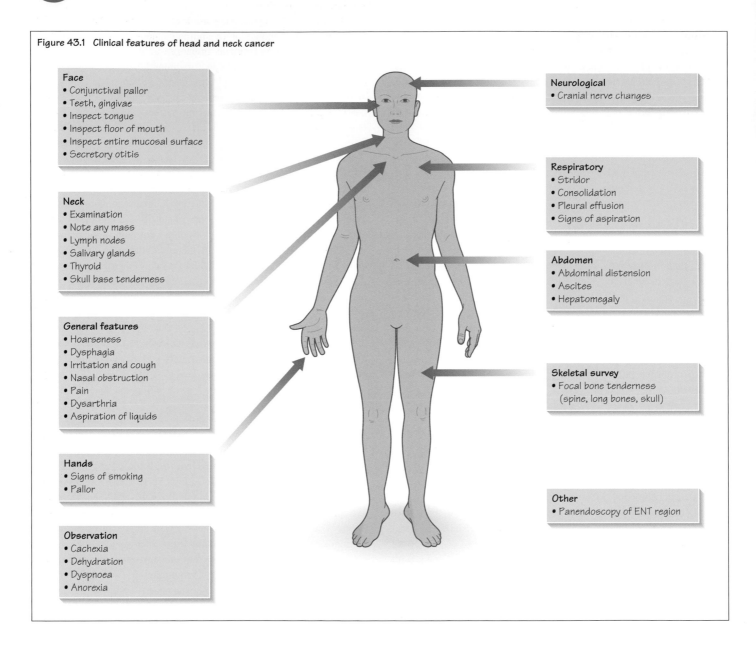

Figure 43.1 Clinical features of head and neck cancer

Face
- Conjunctival pallor
- Teeth, gingivae
- Inspect tongue
- Inspect floor of mouth
- Inspect entire mucosal surface
- Secretory otitis

Neck
- Examination
- Note any mass
- Lymph nodes
- Salivary glands
- Thyroid
- Skull base tenderness

General features
- Hoarseness
- Dysphagia
- Irritation and cough
- Nasal obstruction
- Pain
- Dysarthria
- Aspiration of liquids

Hands
- Signs of smoking
- Pallor

Observation
- Cachexia
- Dehydration
- Dyspnoea
- Anorexia

Neurological
- Cranial nerve changes

Respiratory
- Stridor
- Consolidation
- Pleural effusion
- Signs of aspiration

Abdomen
- Abdominal distension
- Ascites
- Hepatomegaly

Skeletal survey
- Focal bone tenderness
  (spine, long bones, skull)

Other
- Panendoscopy of ENT region

Epidemiology

Head and neck cancer is the sixth most common cancer worldwide and accounts for 4% of all cancer in the UK. It is more common in men (65–90% of cases) than women and incidence increases with age, particularly over 50 years. It can be classified into oral cavity (44%), larynx (31%) and pharynx (25%). These patients have particular problems due to the close proximity of the tumours to important structures in the head and there can be severe social consequences to treatment, e.g. the loss of voice in laryngeal cancer.

Aetiology

The most significant risk factors are smoking (sixfold increased risk), chewing tobacco or betel nuts, and alcohol consumption, particularly spirits which act synergistically with tobacco. Other factors include UV light exposure (lip cancer), viral infections (EBV, HPV), environmental exposure (wood dust, nickel) and radiation (thyroid and salivary gland cancer).

Nasopharyngeal cancer is most common in Southeast Asia and is seen in Arabs and Inuits, but worldwide it is rare. There is a strong association with the major histocompatibility complexes H2B, BW46 and B17. Case-controlled studies in Chinese patients have suggested a link between salted fish consumption and the incidence of nasopharyngeal cancer. Mutations in the *TP53* tumour suppressor gene are recognised and associated with a worse outcome.

Pathophysiology

The majority of head and neck cancers are squamous cell carcinoma (90%), except in nasopharyngeal tumours, which tend to be anaplastic.

Other rare forms include adenoid cystic carcinoma, plasmacytoma, melanoma, sarcoma and lymphoma. Up to 20% of patients can have multiple primary sites at presentation

Clinical examination

Physical examination is the best means for detecting a cancer of the head and neck region. The teeth, gingivae and entire mucosal surface should be inspected. The lymphoid tissue of the tonsillar pillars should be inspected and any asymmetry noted. Tongue mobility should be evaluated. The floor of the mouth, tongue and cheeks should be palpated using a bimanual technique (one gloved finger inside the mouth and the second hand under the mandible). Palpation should be the last step of the examination due to stimulation of the gag reflex. Any suspicious lesions require biopsy.

The neck should be examined, documenting the location of any mass and noting the relationship to major structures, such as the salivary gland, thyroid and carotid sheath. The thyroid should be palpated.

Cancers of the oral cavity present as non-healing ulcers that can be raised, ulcerated, excavated, pigmented, well-demarcated or poorly demarcated and may cause pain. They are often well advanced at presentation and diagnosed by dentists. Investigation is by bimanual palpation. These tumours can be aggressive and invade into the skull base before spreading to lymph nodes.

Laryngeal cancer usually presents with hoarseness. Other symptoms include dysphagia, irritation and coughing. Any patient who presents with hoarseness of >3 weeks should be referred for endoscope. Lymph node involvement is rare due to a poor lymphatic supply to the larynx.

Nasopharyngeal cancer can present with an insidious onset but symptoms include unilateral nasal obstruction, secretory otitis and cranial nerve changes.

Oropharyngeal cancer presents with dysphagia, pain, aspiration of liquids and dysarthria. Due to the anatomy of the oropharynx, lymph nodes can be raised and the tumours are often only visible when the tongue is fully retracted.

Laryngopharyngeal cancer can present with dyspnoea, dysphagia, anorexia, irritation and stridor.

Investigations and staging

Indirect laryngoscopy is used to examine the nasopharynx, hypopharynx and larynx. The vocal cords should be visualised and their mobility evaluated. Mirror examination provides an overall impression of mobility and asymmetry.

Direct laryngoscopy permits inspection of the upper aerodigestive tract, viewing the piriform sinuses, tongue base, pharyngeal walls, epiglottis, arytenoids, and true and false vocal cords.

Endoscopy is useful as 5% of patients with head and neck cancer have a synchronous primary squamous cell cancer of the head and neck, oesophagus or lung, and therefore may require direct laryngoscopy, oesophagoscopy and bronchoscopy.

CT imaging can delineate the extent of disease, the presence of lymph node involvement and can distinguish cystic from solid lesions. Imaging of the chest, abdomen and pelvis may identify the primary site of an occult primary tumour presenting with a lymph node in the neck. CT imaging offers high spatial resolution and can discriminate among fat, muscle, bone and other soft tissues, and it surpasses MRI in the detection of bony erosion.

MRI scanning may provide accurate information regarding the size, location and extent of the tumour, and is better for imaging cancers of the nasopharynx and oropharynx.

Treatment

Oral cancer represents anything from the lip to the anterior two-thirds of the tongue. Treatment of stage 1 tumours is with curative intent and requires radiotherapy or excision depending on the location. Stages 2–4 require the combination of surgery, radiotherapy and chemotherapy. Metastases can be managed by radical dissection of the neck or radiotherapy to the lymph nodes in the neck. Surgery is often the treatment of choice if local recurrence occurs.

Laryngeal cancer can present as a premalignant lesion on the vocal cords, which leads to hoarseness and can be excised endoscopically. For more established cancers radiotherapy is the best treatment as the squamous cells respond well to radiation. In stage 1 and 2 tumours, radiation alone can be curative. Surgery can be used in combination with radiotherapy, but the proximity of the tumour to the vocal cords is important because of the potential for loss of voice. For stage 3 and 4 tumours, radiotherapy with adjuvant chemotherapy is standard.

Nasopharyngeal cancer is treated with radical radiotherapy and/or chemotherapy. Radiotherapy requires precision in the delivery of treatment doses due to the close relationship to the skull base and upper spinal cord. However, prognosis is poor with 5-year survival for stage 1 of 50% and stage 2 of 30%.

Oropharyngeal cancer is treated with surgical excision of the tumour and lymph nodes, followed by radiotherapy. Prognosis is better than for nasopharyngeal cancer as the tumour is more accessible for resection.

Laryngopharyngeal cancer is treated with radical surgery if there is no local spread, followed by radiotherapy, which can be curative for early stage tumours. Radiotherapy is useful for palliation in advanced or recurrent disease. Prognosis is poor, with many patients dying from recurrent disease.

Chemotherapy with carboplatin, paclitaxel and cetuximab, or docetaxel, cisplatin and fluorouracil are used as induction treatments for inoperable, locally advanced squamous cell head & neck cancers.

Prognosis

Prognosis correlates strongly with stage at diagnosis. For many head and neck cancers, survival for patients with stage 1 disease exceeds 80%. For patients with locally advanced disease (stage 3–4) at the time of diagnosis, survival drops below 40%. Development of nodal metastases reduces survival of a small primary tumour by approximately 50%. Involvement of even a single lymph node is associated with a marked decline in survival. Most patients with head and neck cancer have stage 3 or 4 disease at diagnosis.

Despite aggressive primary treatment, the majority of relapses (80%) that occur are locoregional within the head and neck. Distant metastases increase as the disease progresses, and most often involve the lungs, bones and liver. By the time of death, 10–30% of patients will have clinically detected distant metastases.

Table 44.1 TNM staging of thyroid cancer

Classification	Division	Description
T – extent of tumour Categories can contain subdivisions a. for solitary and b. for multiple lesions	Tx	Primary cancer cannot be assessed
	T0	No evidence of cancer
	T1	Tumour <1cm in greatest diameter
	T2	Tumour >1cm but <4cm in greatest diameter
	T3	Tumour >4cm in greatest diameter
	T4	Tumour outside of thyroid capsule can be of any size
N – regional lymph nodes	N0	No cancer in nearby lymph nodes
	N1a	Cancer in lymph nodes close to thyroid in neck (pretracheal, paratracheal, or prelaryngeal)
	N1b	Cancer in other lymph nodes in neck (e.g. cervical, retropharyngeal, superior mediastinal)
M – metastasis	Mx	Cannot be assessed
	M0	No distant metastasis
	M1	Distant metastasis present

Epidemiology

Thyroid cancer is the most common cancer of the endocrine system but is a relatively uncommon malignancy with fewer than 1200 patients registered in the UK every year. The incidence of thyroid nodules in the general population is approximately 5%, with nodules being more common in females than males (2.5:1). The prevalence of thyroid cancer in a solitary nodule or in a multinodular thyroid is 10–20%, increasing with irradiation of the neck.

Papillary, follicular and medullary types are more common in young adults, while the elderly are more likely to develop anaplastic cancer. Geographical regions that were exposed to the Chernobyl disaster or Japanese populations following the atomic bomb detonations have a higher incidence.

Aetiology

Benign thyroid conditions such as enlargement of the thyroid (goitre), inflammation (thyroiditis) and thyroid nodules (adenoma) all increase the risk of thyroid cancer. Radiation exposure is a common predisposing factor and this may be following treatment for childhood cancer or high levels after environmental incidents such as the Chernobyl disaster. Individuals with low levels of iodine who are exposed to radiation are at higher risk of developing thyroid cancer than those with normal levels.

Pathophysiology

Thyroid cancer is classified by morphology from the classical papillary, follicular and anaplastic cancers to Hürthle cell and medullary cell carcinoma and lymphoma. Differentiated (papillary and follicular) thyroid cancers account for more than 90% of cases.

Papillary carcinoma is associated with mutations in *BRAF* (V599E) (40% of cases) and overexpression of cyclin D1 (50%). Furthermore, disruption of the pRb signalling pathway can be seen in papillary and anaplastic cancers due to upregulation of E2F1. Papillary tumours

arise from thyroid follicular cells, are unilateral in most cases and are often multifocal within a single thyroid lobe. They vary in size, from microscopic cancers to large cancers that may invade the thyroid capsule and infiltrate into contiguous structures. Papillary tumours tend to invade the lymphatics, but vascular invasion (and haematogenous spread) is uncommon.

Follicular carcinoma, although mostly encapsulated, commonly has microscopic vascular and capsular invasion. There is usually no lymph node involvement. Follicular carcinoma cancer can be difficult to distinguish from its benign counterpart, follicular adenoma, as the distinction is based on the presence or absence of capsular or vascular invasion, which cannot be evaluated by FNA.

Medullary thyroid cancers represent 10% of all thyroid cancers, arise from the C-cells of the thyroid and secrete calcitonin. About 80% of patients with medullary cancer have a sporadic form, while the remainder have inherited disease. The *RET* proto-oncogene is mutated in almost all patients with MEN 2A and 85% of patients with familial medullary thyroid cancer.

Anaplastic carcinoma represents about 5% of all thyroid cancers; it has a high mitotic rate and is more likely to invade local structures such as lymph nodes.

Clinical presentation

Most patients present with a painless lump in the thyroid or with cervical or supraclavicular lymphadenopathy. Almost all patients are euthyroid. The lump moves with swallowing and tongue protrusion, and is usually firm and non-tender. The presence of a hoarse voice can result from compression of the recurrent laryngeal nerve. Dysphagia and stridor are rare but result from a large tumour compressing the upper airway and oesophagus.

Up to 40% of adults with papillary thyroid cancer may present with regional lymph node metastases. Distant metastases do occur in the lungs, bones and other soft tissues. Children may present with a solitary thyroid nodule, but cervical node involvement is more common in this age group; up to 10% of children and adolescents may have lung involvement at the time of diagnosis.

Sporadic medullary thyroid carcinoma presents as a solitary thyroid mass; metastases to cervical and mediastinal lymph nodes are found in half of patients. Distant metastases to the lungs, liver, bones and adrenal glands occur late in the course of the disease. Secretory diarrhoea, related to calcitonin secretion, can be a clinical feature of advanced medullary thyroid carcinoma. Familial medullary thyroid carcinoma is more likely to present as a bilateral, multifocal process, often with amyloid deposits.

Anaplastic tumours can invade the skin, producing erythema and palpable nodules.

Investigations and staging

Routine investigations include thyroid function tests and thyroid isotope scanning. A thyroid ultrasound can differentiate between solid and cystic lumps and guide fine needle aspiration biopsy, which can provide a cytological diagnosis. Occasionally, the FNA sample is insufficient and a surgical biopsy is required.

Further staging investigations include a chest X-ray and CT scan of the neck and thorax (MRI can be an alternative) (Table 44.1). PET/CT is still under evaluation but can be helpful in assessing response to treatment. Serum calcitonin should be measured in patients with medullary thyroid carcinoma, and thyroglobulin is normally produced by follicular cells of the thyroid and should not be detectable in the serum following thyroidectomy. It may be helpful to follow the course of papillary and follicular thyroid cancer.

Thyroid isotope scans cannot differentiate a benign from a malignant nodule, but can determine the probability based on the functional status of the nodule. Thyroid nodules that concentrate the radioiodine (hot nodules) represent functioning tissue, whereas those that do not concentrate the iodine (cold nodules) are non-functioning and are more likely to be cancer. Most thyroid carcinomas occur in cold nodules but only 10% of cold nodules are carcinomas.

Treatment

After determining the site of cancer and extent of spread, patients should proceed to surgery. For patients with low-risk tumours confined to a single lobe, a subtotal thyroidectomy with removal of the isthmus and affected lobe can be considered. However, for the majority a total thyroidectomy is appropriate. There is no evidence that routine lymph node dissection has any impact on survival, but affected lymph nodes should be removed. Care is required to avoid damage to the parathyroid glands and recurrent laryngeal nerves.

If patients have recurrent or residual disease following surgery, radiotherapy can be considered. This can be given by external beam radiotherapy or radioiodine (follicular or papillary). External beam radiotherapy is more often used for anaplastic and medullary cancers, which do not respond well to radioactive iodine.

Chemotherapy is not used in the treatment of thyroid cancer unless it has metastasised to other parts of the body, and generally it is not very effective.

Following treatment, patients are treated with thyroxine as thyroid replacement, aiming to maintain complete suppression of TSH, which can be a driver for the development of recurrence.

Prognosis

The prognosis for each type of cancer is dependent on the extent of disease at presentation. The involvement of lymph nodes or distant metastasis will significantly lower the survival.

Children have a good prognosis and young adults have a better prognosis than the elderly. Non-invasive cancers have a better outcome compared with those with extracapsular or lymphatic invasion, as well as those with distant metastases.

Tumour type	5-year overall survival (%)
Papillary	80
Follicular	60
Medullary	50
Anaplastic	10

Figure 45.1 Clinical features of bone cancer and sarcoma

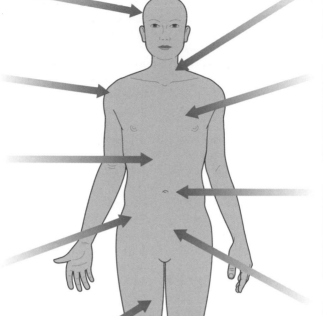

Rhabdomyosarcoma
(sarcoma of skeletal muscle)

Symptoms
• Visible, enlarging mass

Kaposi's sarcoma
(an AIDS-defining illness)
associated with HHV8 infection

Gastrointestinal stromal tissue (GIST)

Symptoms
• Haemoptysis
• Blood in faeces
• Symptoms of anaemia

Chondrosarcoma
(sarcoma of cartilage tissue)
arise from bones in pelvis,
shoulder, and limbs

Symptoms
• Painful bony swellings
• Pathological fractures

Liposarcoma
(sarcoma of fat tissue)

Symptoms
• Enlarging deep-seated mass in
  soft tissue
• Found in the thigh or in the
  retroperitoneum

Angiosarcoma
(sarcoma of blood vessels)

Symptoms
• Painful swelling

Lung metastasis

Symptoms
• Cough
• Breathlessness
• Haemoptysis
• Chest pain

Gastric leiomyosarcoma
(sarcoma of smooth muscle cells)

Symptoms
• Early satiety
• Weight loss
• Abdominal pain

Endometrial stromal sarcoma
(sarcoma of connective tissue cells)

Symptoms
• Passing blood PV
• Low abdominal pain

Osteosarcoma
(sarcoma of bone)

Symptoms
• Painful bony swelling
• Overlying erythema
• Pathological fractures (rare)

Table 45.1 Clinical features of soft tissue sarcoma

Tumour	Age (years)	Commonest sites	Primary therapy	5-year overall survival (%)
Alveolar rhabdomyosarcoma	10–20	Thigh	Neoadjuvant chemoradiation and surgery	60
Angiosarcoma	50–70	Skin, superficial soft tissues	Wide excision and adjuvant radiation	15
Embryonal rhabdomyosarcoma	0–10	Head and neck, genitourinary (botyroid)	Neoadjuvant chemoradiation and surgery	40
Fibrosarcoma	20–50	Thigh, arm, head and neck	Wide excision and adjuvant radiation	90 (well diff.) 50 (poorly diff.)
Leiomyosarcoma	45–65	Retroperitoneal, uterine	Wide excision and adjuvant radiation	40
Liposarcoma	40–60	Thigh, head and neck (rarely arise from lipoma)	Wide excision and adjuvant radiation	66 (myxoid) 10 (pleomorphic)
Pleomorphic rhabdomyosarcoma	40–70	Thigh, upper arm	Wide excision and adjuvant radiation	10
Synovial sarcoma	20–40	Leg	Wide excision and adjuvant radiation	40

Epidemiology

Sarcomas are tumours of the body's supportive connective tissue and can arise from bone, muscle, cartilage, tendon, fat, or synovial tissue. They account for less than 1% of all cancers. Ewing's sarcoma and osteosarcoma develop primarily in children and adolescents, and occurrence appears to correlate with the growth spurt.

Soft tissue sarcomas are rare in adults, but account for approximately 6% of all childhood cancers.

Aetiology

For the majority of **bone sarcomas** no specific aetiology has been established, although predisposing factors have been identified. Children with familial retinoblastoma have a 13q chromosome deletion and an increased incidence of osteosarcoma (see Chapter 8). Radiation-associated sarcomas develop within a radiation field usually after a latent period of at least 3 years and the majority are osteosarcoma. Alkylating agents and anthracyclines have been implicated in the development of second malignancies, particularly osteosarcoma. In adults, osteosarcoma is often associated with an underlying bone abnormality such as Paget's disease, fibrous dysplasia, or where the bone has been irradiated previously.

For **soft tissue sarcomas**, there is a genetic association with neurofibromatosis type 1, hereditary retinoblastoma and Li–Fraumeni syndrome. Previous radiation therapy increases the risk of developing sarcoma and exposure to chemicals such as vinyl chloride monomer, dioxin, or herbicides are risk factors for developing sarcomas (see Chapter 3).

Ewing's sarcoma typically arises from the axial skeleton and is associated with the t(11;22) chromosomal translocation. This chromosomal alteration juxtaposes the *EWS* and *FLI1* genes, producing a hybrid transcript that is able to act as a master regulatory protein.

Clinical presentation

Most osteosarcomas occur in the metaphyseal region of growing long bones, such as the distal femur, proximal tibia and proximal humerus. Ewing's sarcoma is classically described as a diaphyseal lesion but may arise from any region within an involved long bone. It commonly arises in the flat bones of the pelvis and scapula. Primary bone tumours of any histological subtype are extremely rare in the spine and sacrum (Table 43.1).

Bone sarcomas typically present with localised pain, which initially is insidious and transient, but worsens progressively. Localised soft tissue swelling, with or without associated warmth and erythema, may be present. Joint effusions may be detectable, and range of movement of the adjacent joints may be limited and painful. Movement or weight bearing of the involved extremity may exacerbate local symptoms. Interestingly, regional lymph nodes are only rarely involved. Constitutional symptoms are rare; however, fever, malaise and weight loss can be seen with Ewing's sarcoma.

Soft tissue sarcomas usually present with painless soft tissue swelling. However, if located within a body cavity, they may cause pain or exert pressure on nearby structures. Gastrointestinal stromal tissue (GIST) tumours can cause bleeding and may present as haematemesis, blood in faeces, or even anaemia. Uterine sarcoma can present with vaginal bleeding or lower abdominal pain.

Investigations and staging

Although many **bone sarcomas** are visible on plain X-rays, MRI is required to assess the extent of the lesions as well as the relationship of tumours to nearby structures such as nerves, blood vessels and joints. Intramedullary tumour extent and presence of skip metastases within the bone are best demonstrated by MRI. An isotope bone scan may be helpful for detecting distant osseous metastases. There are no useful tumour markers but alkaline phosphatase and LDH may be raised in some cases. A biopsy is required and should be undertaken by a specialist orthopaedic oncologist to avoid seeding of the needle tract, which could compromise future curative therapy.

MRI is the investigation of choice for **soft tissue sarcomas**. A chest X-ray or chest CT can identify lung metastasis, as these tumours will metastasise by blood-borne spread to the lung. Biopsy for histology is required and can be image-guided or open during resection.

Patients with Ewing's sarcoma require a biopsy as well as a bone marrow aspirate and trephine biopsy from distant sites to check for metastasis. Patients are commonly anaemic, with elevated ESR, CRP and LDH.

Treatment

Bone sarcomas should be considered for limb-sparing surgery with endoprosthetic replacement of the resected bone rather than amputation. If surgery is combined with adjuvant or neoadjuvant chemotherapy, a positive response to chemotherapy is a good prognostic factor. The specialist surgeon must ensure that the entire local tumour is removed, with wide clear margins, and approximately 95% of osteosarcoma surgery is limb sparing. Muscle can be reconstructed using transfers from other parts of the body, with the goal of producing a functional limb. Radiotherapy can be used for non-resectable tumours, or where the excision margins are not satisfactory, or for palliation of bone metastasis. Patients with metastatic disease can be treated with palliative chemotherapy, radiotherapy, or amputation to improve symptom control.

Patients with **soft tissue sarcomas** require surgery aimed at complete excision of the tumour with clear margins. This may require en bloc dissection with removal of the muscular compartments, which gives the lowest risk of local recurrence. Limb amputation is necessary in 5% of cases. Adjuvant or neoadjuvant chemotherapy or radiotherapy are of limited use.

GIST tumours respond to the tyrosine kinase inhibitor imatinib and treatment may significantly increase the median survival time in patients with disease unresponsive to conventional chemotherapy.

Treatment of Ewing's sarcoma requires a multidisciplinary approach and usually consists of chemotherapy followed by surgical excision and then further chemotherapy (see Chapter 53).

Prognosis

Bone sarcomas have a 5-year survival of 60–70% for localised disease and 10–30% for metastatic disease.

Soft tissue sarcomas have a 5-year survival of 70% and careful monitoring is required, as patients with solitary pulmonary metastasis can be cured by surgical resection. Ewing's sarcoma has a 5-year survival of 55–60% for localised disease and 10–20% for metastatic disease.

Table 46.1 The ABCDE rule for examining suspicious naevii

A – Asymmetry	Melanomas are usually asymmetrical, compared with a majority of non-melanoma lesions that are symmetrical
B – Border	Normal naevii can have a well-defined border. Dysplastic naevii and melanomas usually have ill-defined borders
C – Colour	Melanomas can have a variety of colours present, not a uniform colour like a normal naevii
D – Diameter	If diameter has increased, this is a suspicious sign. Melanomas when first seen often have a diameter greater than 7mm
E – Elevation	Melanomas can feel elevated to the touch; this is a sign of invasion and more advanced disease

Table 46.2 Clinicopathological features of common forms of melanoma

Type	Location	Age (median)	Gender and race	Edge	Colour	Frequency
Superficial spreading	All body surfaces, particularly legs	56 years	White females	Palpable, irregular	Brown, black, grey or pink, central or halo depigmentation	50%
Nodular	All body surfaces	49 years	White males	Palpable	Uniform bluish black	30%
Lentigo maligna	Sun-exposed especially head and neck	70 years	White females	Flat, irregular	Shades of brown or black, hypopigmentation	15%
Acral lentigenous	Palms, soles and mucous membranes	61 years	Black males	Palpable, irregular nodule	Black, irregularly coloured	5%

Table 46.3 British Association of Dermatologists' guidelines for the excision margins for melanoma

Breslow thickness	Excision margin
In situ	5mm
<1mm	1cm
1.01–2mm	1–2cm
2.01–4mm	2–3cm
>4mm	3cm

Epidemiology

Skin cancer is one of the most commonly diagnosed cancers in the UK, with more than 86 000 cases diagnosed annually. There are two major types of skin cancer: melanoma and non-melanoma.

Aetiology

The main risk factor for both types is increased exposure to ultraviolet (UV) radiation. Short periods of intense sun exposure, which can result in sunburn, will increase the risk of melanoma. Chronic exposure increases the risk of non-melanoma skin cancers. Other factors such as skin type, family history and a previous history of skin cancer are important. Patients who have had a renal transplant have a 33-fold increased risk of non-melanoma skin cancer due to immunosuppressive therapy, and have a higher risk of melanoma.

Non-melanoma skin cancer
Basal cell carcinoma

This is the most common skin cancer and arises from the basal cell layer of the skin. The majority occur in sun-exposed areas of the skin. They rarely metastasise but can ulcerate and invade locally, which if left untreated can cause extensive damage, particularly around the ears, nose and eyes. This gave them the name 'rodent ulcer'.

Basal cell carcinomas (BCC) usually have a pearly rolled edge, central ulceration and telengiectasia on the surface, although not all present this way. Other features include a persistent, non-healing sore, an erythematous scaly plaque (which may have been misdiagnosed as eczema or psoriasis), or a waxy papule with poorly defined borders.

Diagnosis is usually made on the visual appearance and biopsy is required to confirm the histological subtype.

Early treatment is vital due to the risk of invasion, and approaches can be surgical or non-surgical. Surgical treatment involves excision, although electrocautery, which is used to destroy the tumour before it is scrapped away using curettage, is becoming popular. Moh's micrographic surgery is an alternative treatment used for higher-risk patients or more aggressive histological subtypes. Moh's surgery involves the removal of the tumour in stages, with each sample checked by a histologist before further removal occurs. This has a high success rate, but is a long procedure and requires specialist equipment. Cryotherapy can be used for small, low-risk lesions. Other non-surgical approaches involve the use of topical imiquimod or fluorouracil, photodynamic therapy, or radiotherapy.

Prognosis is good with low mortality, but patients with BCC are at increased risk of developing more BCCs, in addition to squamous cell carcinoma and melanoma.

Squamous cell carcinoma

Squamous cell carcinoma (SCC) arises from the keratinising cells of the epidermis and occurs in sun-exposed areas due to the effects of UV radiation. In addition, industrial chemicals and tobacco chewing are important risk factors, along with immunosupresssion. These lesions arise on top of pre-malignant changes such as actinic (solar) keratosis, Bowen's disease (in-situ SCC) and leukoplakia. SCC can be present in areas of chronic ulceration (Marjolin's ulcer).

An SCC can present as an ulcerated nodule with surrounding erythema and can bleed easily when traumatised. These cancers can metastasise and therefore patients require careful examination of the regional lymph nodes. If there is involvement of the ear, lip, oral cavity, tongue, or genitalia, special management is required and the patient should be referred to an appropriate specialist.

Diagnosis and management are similar to that for BCC, although patients usually require CT imaging for the staging of their tumour. A surgical excision is preferred where the lesion is removed to deep fat with a 4 mm margin (if the lesion is <1 cm in size). Other non-surgical options can be considered, but all patients should be referred to the specialist skin cancer multidisciplinary team.

Prognosis is variable, with the depth of invasion of the primary tumour corresponding to the risk of metastases and overall survival. Patients with metastatic disease have a 30% 5-year survival. Education is the key to prevention, with efforts to minimise exposure to UV radiation the key principle.

Melanoma

Melanocytes are found in the basal cell layer of the epidermis, and produce melanin, a pigment responsible for skin colour. Non-malignant melanocytic growth produces benign melanocytic naevi, or lentigines (moles and freckles). Exposure of these lesions to UV radiation can cause malignant change, producing a melanoma. Risk factors include sun exposure, skin pigmentation, family history and history of dysplastic naevii.

Melanomas can occur anywhere on the skin surface and can be asymptomatic or present with bleeding and itching. A key sign is a changing naevus, which can be evaluated using the ABCDE rule (Table 46.1). If a naevus fits any of these criteria then referral to a specialist is essential.

A biopsy may confirm malignant melanoma or lentigo maligna, an irregularly pigmented lesion that spreads laterally and is similar to an in-situ cancer. The common types of melanoma are outlined in Table 46.2. The biopsy determines the Breslow thickness, a measure of how deep the melanoma has spread downwards, and this strongly relates to prognosis. CT imaging is used to determine the extent of spread.

The primary treatment is wide local excision with varying excision margins according to the Breslow thickness (Table 46.3). Further surgery with lymph node dissection may be required.

The prognosis for metastatic melanoma is poor and patients often have multiple sites of involvement. Treatment depends on patient fitness and disease site, but patients are usually treated with chemotherapy such as dacarbazine or biological agents such as ipilimumab. Radiotherapy is often used after surgical resection for patients with locally or regionally advanced melanoma or for patients with unresectable distant metastases. It may reduce the rate of local recurrence but does not prolong survival. Radiotherapy is useful for palliation, although often has a limited effect.

About 60% of melanomas contain a mutation in the *BRAF* gene and specific inhibitors such as vemurafenib can produce significant tumour regressions in patients with a *BRAF* gene mutation.

When there is distant metastasis, melanoma is considered incurable and the 5-year survival rate is less than 10%. The median survival is 6–12 months. Metastases to skin and lungs have a better prognosis, while metastases to brain, bone and liver have a worse prognosis.

Figure 47.1 Clinical features of cancer of the central nervous system

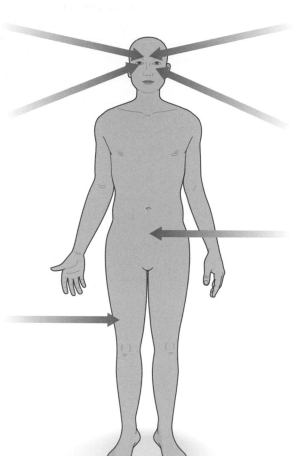

Olfactory groove tumour
- Anosmia
- Visual loss
- Frontal lobe syndrome
- Papilloedema

Sella turcica tumour
- Visual field loss

Parasagital falx tumour
- Progressive spastic weakness
- Progressive numbness of legs

General
- Confusion
- Cognitive dysfunction
- Personality changes
- Seizures
- Headache
- Cushingoid features (steroids)

Posterior fossa tumour
- Ataxic gait
- Cranial neuropathies (V, VII, VIII, IX, X)
- Cerebellopontine angle
- Suboccipital pain
- Hydrocephalus
- Ispilateral arm and leg weakness

Sphenoid wing tumour
- Exophthalmos and visual loss
- Temporal bone swelling
- Skull deformity (lateral)
- Cavernous sinus syndrome

Spinal axis tumour
- Bilateral symmetrical UMN signs
- Bone tenderness
- Urinary retention
- Sensorimotor dysfunction
- Root infiltration
- Radicular pain
- Syringomyelia

Look for
- Primary site of carcinoma
- Lymphoma
- Sarcoma

Exclude metastasis especially from
- Lung
- Breast
- Skin (melanoma)
- Kidney

Table 47.1 Types of cancer of the central nervous system

Gliomas (50% of brain tumours) include	Non-glial brain tumours include
• **Grade I** (non-infiltrating pilocytic astrocytoma)	• **Meningiomas** (most common, 15% of non-glial tumours)
• **Grade II** (well to moderately differentiated astrocytoma)	• **Pineal parenchymal tumours**
• **Grade III** (anaplastic astrocytoma)	• **Extragonal germ cell tumours**
• **Grade IV** (glioblastoma multiforme)	• **Craniopharyngiomas**
• **Other glial tumours**	• **Choroid plexus tumours**
– **Ependymomas** that arise from ependymal cells lining usually the fourth ventricle	• **Primary cerebral non-Hodgkin's lymphoma**
	Primary spinal cord tumours include
– **Oligodendrogliomas** that arise from oligodendroglia	• **Schwannomas** (29%)
– **Medulloblastomas** are tumours of childhood, usually arising in the cerebellum and may be related to primitive neuroectodermal tumours elsewhere in central nervous system (CNS)	• **Extradural meningiomas** (26%)
	• **Intramedullary ependymomas** (13%)
	• **Astrocytomas** (13%)

Epidemiology

Brain tumours account for 2–5% of all cancers and 2% of cancer deaths. Metastases to the brain are more common than primary brain tumours and often arise from cancers of the lung, breast, skin (melanoma) and kidney. Furthermore, nasopharyngeal cancers can extend directly through the foramina of the skull and involve the brain. Meningeal metastases occur with systemic spread from leukaemia, lymphoma, breast cancer and small-cell lung cancer, and from local extension of medulloblastoma and ependymal gliomas. Fewer than 20% of CNS tumours occur in the spinal cord. The types of cancer of the CNS are outlined in Table 47.1.

Aetiology

The cause of most adult brain tumours is not known. Several inherited phakomatoses are associated with brain tumours that tend to occur in children or young adults and include:
- tuberous sclerosis (gliomas, ependymomas);
- Li–Fraumeni syndrome (glioma);
- Turcot syndrome (gliomas);
- neurofibromatosis type I (cranial and root schwannomas, meningiomas, ependymomas, optic gliomas);
- von Hippel–Lindau disease (cerebellar and retinal haemangioblastoma);
- Gorlin's basal naevus syndrome (medulloblastoma).

Clinical presentation
Glial tumours

General symptoms include those produced by mass effect; increased intracranial pressure, oedema, midline shift and herniation can all produce a progressive altered mental state, personality changes, headaches, seizures and papilloedema. Focal symptoms depend on the location of the tumour. Fewer than 10% of primary seizures are due to tumours and only 20% of supratentorial tumours present with seizures.

Meningioma

These tumours present as a slowly growing mass that can produce headache, seizures, motor and sensory disturbance, and depending on their site, cranial neuropathies. Meningiomas can produce characteristic changes on plain skull radiographs with bone erosion, calcification and hyperostosis. They are more common in women.

Spinal axis tumours

The frequency of tumour sites is 70% thoracic, 20% lumbosacral and 10% cervical, most commonly from cancer of the breast, lung, or prostate, or from sarcoma or lymphoma. These tumours present with:
- sensorimotor dysfunction due to cord compression (the most common, and due to metastasis);
- radicular symptoms due to root infiltration (often local extension of a tumour);
- syringomyelia symptoms due to intramedullary tumours causing central destruction (can be primary tumours within the CNS).

Investigations and staging

MRI with gadolinium enhancement is the imaging of choice. Positron emission tomography (PET) may help to differentiate tumour recurrence from radiation necrosis. A biopsy is required to confirm the diagnosis, although occasionally diagnosis on clinical evidence is made if biopsy is hazardous (e.g. brainstem gliomas). Staging is not applicable to most primary brain tumours as they are locally invasive and do not spread to regional lymph nodes or distant organs.

Treatment

Rarely, gliomas are curable by surgery with or without radiotherapy, but the majority require surgery, radiotherapy and chemotherapy. Surgical removal should be as complete as possible within the constraints of preserving neurological function.

Radiotherapy can increase the cure rate or prolong disease-free survival in high-grade gliomas and may produce symptomatic improvement in patients with low-grade gliomas who relapse after initial therapy with surgery alone.

Chemotherapy (nitrosourea-based or temozolomide) may prolong disease-free survival in patients with oligodendrogliomas and high-grade gliomas, although the toxicity may be limiting.

Meningiomas require surgical resection, which can be repeated if the tumour relapses. Radiotherapy reduces the relapse rate and should be considered for high-grade meningiomas or incompletely resected tumours. Relapse rates are 7% at 5 years if completely resected and 35–60% if incompletely resected.

Complications

Early complications of radiotherapy (first 3–4 months) are due to reversible damage to myelin-producing oligodendrocytes that recover spontaneously after 3–6 months. It can produce somnolence or exacerbation of existing symptoms in the brain and Lhermitte's sign (shooting numbness or paraesthesia precipitated by neck flexion) in the spinal cord.

Late complications include irreversible radiation necrosis due to blood vessel damage. This may mimic disease recurrence and correlates with radiation dose, occurring in up to 15% of patients with, the highest frequency in children receiving chemotherapy.

Prognosis

Prognostic factors include histology, grade and size of tumour, age and performance status of patient, and duration of symptoms. Median survival of anaplastic astrocytoma is 18 months; glioblastoma multiforme is 10–12 months. The prognosis of glioma deteriorates with increasing grade of tumour. Meningiomas, if completely resected, are usually cured with a median survival of greater than 10 years.

Five-year survival rates of adult brain tumours	
Tumour	5-year overall survival (%)
Grade I glioma (cerebellar)	90–100
Grade I glioma (all sites)	50–60
Grade II (astrocytoma)	16–46
Grade III (anaplastic astrocytoma)	10–30
Grade IV (glioblastoma multiforme)	1–10
Oligodendroglioma	50–80
Meningioma	70–80

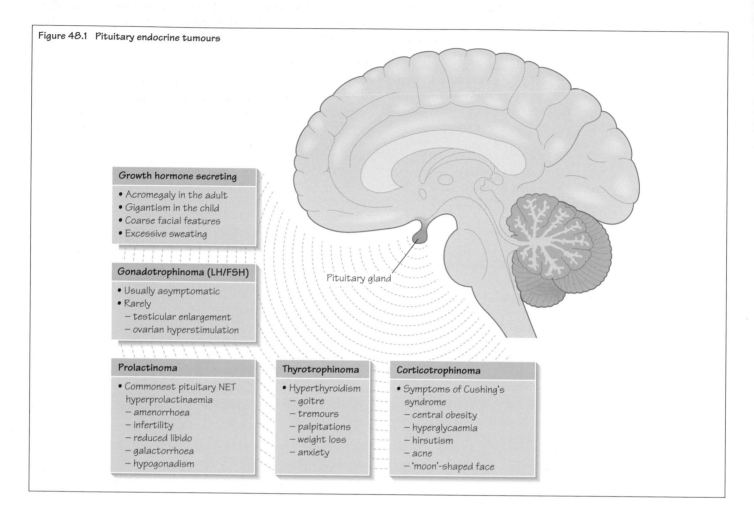

Figure 48.1 Pituitary endocrine tumours

Growth hormone secreting
- Acromegaly in the adult
- Gigantism in the child
- Coarse facial features
- Excessive sweating

Gonadotrophinoma (LH/FSH)
- Usually asymptomatic
- Rarely
  - testicular enlargement
  - ovarian hyperstimulation

Pituitary gland

Prolactinoma
- Commonest pituitary NET hyperprolactinaemia
  - amenorrhoea
  - infertility
  - reduced libido
  - galactorrhoea
  - hypogonadism

Thyrotrophinoma
- Hyperthyroidism
  - goitre
  - tremours
  - palpitations
  - weight loss
  - anxiety

Corticotrophinoma
- Symptoms of Cushing's syndrome
  - central obesity
  - hyperglycaemia
  - hirsutism
  - acne
  - 'moon'-shaped face

Neuroendocrine tumours (NETs) are slow growing and may secrete bioactive peptides and hormones. They can arise anywhere in the body, although most commonly in the gastrointestinal tract, lungs, pancreas, pituitary (see Figure 48.1), parathyroid and thyroid. They are usually benign with symptoms resulting from hormone production, but malignant transformation can result.

NETs may be generally categorised by site of origin, histological appearance, embryological origin, or grade of the tumour. There is dispute as to a single classification system, but currently site of origin is used, with detail given as to the humoral capabilities of the tumour.

Functioning NETs produce bioactive substances that produce clinical symptoms, but if originating within the gastrointestinal tract they require the presence of liver metastasis to produce symptoms due to the effect of first-pass metabolism. Non-functioning NETs may secrete bioactive substances but often at subclinical levels and therefore are not associated with a particular hormonal syndrome. The most common symptoms are due to the physical effects of the tumour and non-specific symptoms may be present.

Argentaffin and hormone secretion

NETs from a particular anatomical origin often show similar behaviour as a group, such as tumours arising in the foregut (includes oesophagus, stomach, duodenum, liver, pancreas, thymus, lung), midgut (bowel from jejunum to transverse colon, appendix) and hindgut (descending colon, sigmoid, rectum).

- **Foregut NETs** are argentaffin negative. Despite low serotonin content, they often secrete 5-hydroxytryptophan (5-HTP), histamine and several polypeptide hormones. There may be associated atypical carcinoid syndrome, acromegaly, Cushing's disease, other endocrine disorders, telangiectasia, or hypertrophy of the skin in the face and upper neck. These tumours can metastasise to bone.
- **Midgut NETs** are argentaffin positive, producing high levels of serotonin (5-HT), kinins, prostaglandins, substance P and other vasoactive peptides, and occasionally ACTH. Bone metastasis is uncommon.
- **Hindgut NETs** are argentaffin negative and rarely secrete 5-HT, 5-HTP, or any other vasoactive peptides. Bone metastases are common.

Carcinoid tumours

These tumours are derived from enterochromaffin cells and usually release serotonin; 90% arise in the appendix and ileum. They are associated with the carcinoid syndrome: flushing, wheeze, diarrhoea, hypotension, telangectasia, bronchoconstriction and heart disease. This is due to high serotonin levels, although carcinoid syndrome is present in only 10% of patients as it requires liver metastases to bypass the effects of first-pass metabolism. An atypical carcinoid syndrome exists, which is related to the serotonin precursor 5-HTP.

Specific investigations include 5-hydroxyindoleacetic acid in a 24-hour urine collection and plasma tachykinins. Somatostatin receptor scintigraphy (octreoscan) is the standard imaging technique. Radioisotope-labelled ocreotide is injected intravenously and binds with high affinity to somatostatin receptors 2 and 5, which are commonly found in NETs. This allows the location of tumours to be visualised and mIBG (meta-iodobenzylguanidine) can be used in a similar way.

Management is primarily with surgery, which can produce long remission periods following complete resection of the tumour and affected local lymph nodes. Optimal debulking should be performed if the patient is fit for surgery, as 70–90% of patients have a significant improvement in symptoms following resection.

Somatostatin analogues can control symptoms and prevent progression where complete resection is impossible or prior to surgical management. Somatostatin inhibits hormone secretion by binding to the somatostatin receptor subtypes located on neuroendocrine cells. It is not clinically useful due to a short half-life, so analogues such as ocreotide and lanreotide are used.

While chemotherapy has no significant effect in typical disease, it may be used in widely metastatic or high-grade NETs, or those not responsive to conventional treatment. Chemotherapy is used more commonly in pancreatic NETs, which have better response rates.

Targeted radiotherapy can be used to relieve pain from bone metastases, with mIBG or ocreotide used to deliver radioisotope radiation therapy.

Newer treatments include mTOR inhibitors, which inhibit a regulator of protein synthesis that is seen in several forms of NET.

Gastroenteropancreatic NETs

Insulinoma

Insulinoma is an insulin-secreting tumour comprised of beta islet cells and is usually benign. Normal feedback mechanisms for the maintenance of normoglycaemia are ineffective, resulting in hypoglycaemia, which produces symptoms of diplopia, blurred vision, confusion, seizures, coma, weakness, sweating, tremor, tachycardia, palpitations and anxiety. Whipples triad can be a feature, and includes symptoms of hypoglycaemia, hypoglycaemia measured during symptoms and symptom relief following administration of glucose.

A drug history should be taken because sulfonylureas stimulate insulin release and accidental administration of the wrong insulin dose may cause these symptoms. Endogenous insulin breaks down into insulin and C-peptide, whereas C-peptide is absent with exongenous insulin, allowing differentiation between potential causes.

Gastrinoma

These are rare tumours associated with excess gastrin secretion that can result in gastric and duodenal ulceration. Gastrinoma should be suspected in patients with multiple or atypical ulceration.

Glucagonoma

These are tumours formed of alpha islet cells in the pancreas and result in increased plasma glucagon levels. Clinical features include diabetes, dermatitis (necrolytic migratory erythema), deep vein thrombosis and depression.

VIPoma

These tumours secrete vasoactive intestinal polypeptide (VIP), which stimulates secretion and inhibits reabsroption of water, potassium, sodium and chloride in the small bowel. Patients present with dehydration, hypokalaemia and achlorhydria associated with high-volume, odourless diarrhoea that persists despite fasting. The majority are metastatic at the time of diagnosis and fasting plasma VIP is measured for diagnosis.

Somatostatinoma

This rare NET results in the inhibition of almost all gastric hormones. Patients present late, particularly as the typical presentation is vague abdominal discomfort. In 10% of patients there is a syndrome of gallstones, steatorrhoea, mild diabetes, weight loss and reduced stomach acid.

Phaeochromocytoma

These are quite rare and usually benign catecholamine-releasing tumours that occur in the medulla of the adrenal glands. They are associated with multiple endocrine neoplasia type 2 (MEN 2) and a careful family history should be taken.

Presentation may be incidental, with intermittent severe hypertension or unresponsive essential hypertension. Patients may complain of headaches, tachycardia, palpitations, sweating, pallor and tremor as a result of increased levels of circulating catecholamines such as adrenaline.

Urine and plasma catecholamines are measured for diagnosis and to monitor response to treatment, and these patients usually require antihypertensive therapy.

Serum tumour markers

Symptoms from secreted hormones may prompt assessment of the corresponding hormones in serum or their associated urinary products. These can be used to assist diagnosis or for response assessment following treatment. There are only a limited range of useful markers and the most important are:

- chromogranin A (CgA);
- urine 5-hydroxyindoleacetic acid (5-HIAA);
- neuron-specific enolase (NSE, gamma-gamma dimer);
- synaptophysin (P38).

Newer markers include N-terminally truncated variant of Hsp70, which is present in NETs but absent in normal pancreatic islets. High levels of CDX2, a homeobox gene product essential for intestinal development and differentiation, is seen in intestinal NETs. Neuroendocrine secretory protein-55, a member of the chromogranin family, is seen in pancreatic endocrine tumours but not intestinal.

Figure 49.1   Clinical features of leukaemia

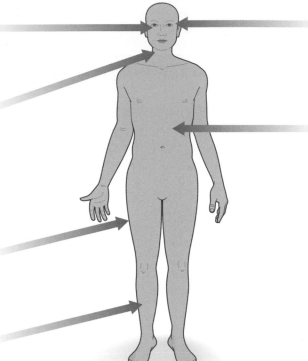

Face
- Conjunctival pallor
- Retinal haemorrhage
- Pallor of mucous membranes
- Gum hypertrophy (AML)

Lymph nodes
- Usually symmetrical
- Mobile, non-tender
- Axilla
- Supraclavicular
- Cervical
- Antecubital
- Mediastinal
  (80% of T-cell ALL)

Skin
- Petichae
- Ecchymosis
- Palmar crease pallor
- Skin involvement (AML)

Musculoskeletal
- Bone pain

Neurological
- Cranial nerve palsies
- Diplopia
- Leptomeningeal infiltration
- Focal neurological signs
- Weakness

Abdomen
- Early satiety
- Hepatomegaly
- Splenomegaly
  (massive in CLL)
- Hepatosplenomegaly
  (massive in CML)
- Chloroma in small bowel
- Mesenteric mass

Other
- Anaemia
- Pancytopenia
- Thrombocytopenia
- Weight loss (CLL)
- Night sweats (CLL)
- Malaise
- Fatigue

Table 49.1   WHO classification of acute myeloid leukaemia

Acute myeloid leukaemia with recurrent genetic abnormalities	• Acute myeloid leukaemia with t(8;21)(q22;q22), (AML1/ETO) • Acute myeloid leukaemia with abnormal bone marrow eosinophils and inv(16)(p13q22) or t(16;16)(p13;q22), (CBFβ/MYH11) • Acute promyelocytic leukaemia with t(15;17)(q22;q12), (PML/RARα) and variants • Acute myeloid leukaemia with 11q23 (MLL) abnormalities
Acute myeloid leukaemia with multilineage dysplasia	• Following MDS or MDS/MPD • Without antecedent MDS or MDS/MPD, but with dysplasia in at least 50% of cells in two or more myeloid lineages
Acute myeloid leukaemia and myelodysplastic syndromes, therapy-related	• Alkylating agent/radiation-related type • Topoisomerase II inhibitor-related type (some may be lymphoid) • Others
Acute myeloid leukaemia, not otherwise categorised	• Acute myeloid leukaemia, minimally differentiated • Acute myeloid leukaemia without maturation • Acute myeloid leukaemia with maturation • Acute myelomonocytic leukaemia • Acute monoblastic/acute monocytic leukaemia • Acute erythroid leukaemia (erythroid/myeloid and pure erythroleukaemia) • Acute megakaryoblastic leukaemia • Acute basophilic leukaemia • Acute panmyelosis with myelofibrosis • Myeloid sarcoma

Epidemiology and pathogenesis

Leukaemias are categorised by cell lineage into four broad groups. In **acute lymphoblastic leukaemia (ALL)**, 60% of cases are in children, with a peak incidence in the first 5 years of life, and drop until age 60, when a second peak emerges. In comparison, **acute myeloid leukaemia (AML)** is less common in children (20%) but is more common in those over the age of 60. The incidence of both AML and ALL is slightly higher in males than females.

In **chronic myeloid leukaemia (CML)**, the median age at presentation is 50–60 years but is seen in all age groups. **Chronic lymphoid leukaemia (CLL)** is the most common leukaemia in adults in Western Europe, accounting for 25% of all leukaemias.

Leukaemia arises from a monoclonal origin where cellular clones have an advantage over normal haematological cells. More than 90% of CML cases and a subset of ALL are associated with a reciprocal translocation between chromosomes 9 and 22, which creates a fusion gene from a juxtaposition of the *BCR* and *ABL* genes, manifesting as the Philadelphia chromosome.

There is an increased incidence of AML and myelodysplasia seen in persons with prolonged exposure to benzene and petroleum products. Prior chemotherapy with alkylating agents (e.g. cyclophosphamide, melphalan) has been associated with the development of AML, usually within 3–5 years of exposure and often preceded by a myelodysplastic phase. An increased incidence of AML is associated with Down syndrome, Bloom syndrome, Fanconi anaemia and ataxia-telangiectasia. AML arising from myelodysplastic syndromes is often the most resistant to treatment and has a worse prognosis.

Clinical presentation

Leukaemia manifests with symptoms related to its impact on normal haematopoiesis, such as easy fatigability, bruising, bleeding from mucosal surfaces, fever and infection. Patients with very high white cell counts may develop hyperviscosity syndrome, presenting with priapism, tinnitus, stupor, retinal haemorrhages and CVA.

Mild hepatosplenomegaly and lymphadenopathy are common, particularly in childhood ALL. Massive hepatosplenomegaly is unusual in acute leukaemias and mediastinal lymphadenopathy is seen in 80% of cases of T-cell ALL, but is less common in other ALLs and is rare in AML. Bone pain is common in children with ALL (40–50%) but is less common in adults (5–10%).

Physical findings in AML are usually minimal; pallor, ecchymoses or petechiae, retinal haemorrhages, gingival hypertrophy and cutaneous involvement are more common with monocytic variants. Visceral involvement is rare, occurring as an initial manifestation of AML (<5% of cases), but may be more frequent during relapses.

In CLL, 20% of patients are asymptomatic with diagnosis discovered on a routine blood examination. In CML, splenomegaly is found in 30% and hepatomegaly in 10–40% of cases. CLL is associated with an increased risk of infection, whereas in CML the risk of infection is only during the accelerated phase.

Investigations and classification

The diagnosis of leukaemia requires examination of the peripheral blood and bone marrow. In patients with ALL a lumbar puncture is required to identify CNS infiltration. Immunophenotyping is performed in suspected ALL to identify B- and T-cell markers, as approximately 75% of cases are B cell. Marrow involvement of >25% lymphoblasts is used as the demarcation line between ALL and lymphoblastic lymphoma, in which the preponderance of tumour bulk is in nodal structures.

Molecular and cytogenetic abnormalities can provide important prognostic information. In AML, the t(8;21) translocation produces the fusion gene of *AML1/ETO*, which is associated with a good prognosis. The WHO classification is used for AML.

The Philadelphia chromosome t(9;22) translocation is found in 5% of childhood and 25% of adult ALL and confers a poor prognosis. T-cell ALL is frequently associated with translocations of T-cell receptor genes on chromosome 14q11 or chromosome 7q34 with other gene partners. T-cell ALL had been associated with a poor prognosis when treated with conventional ALL regimens but responds better to more aggressive antimetabolite therapy. Mature B-cell ALL, also known as Burkitt-cell leukaemia, is associated with translocations of the c-myc gene on chromosome 8 and the immunoglobulin heavy-chain gene on chromosome 14q32 in 80% of cases, or with the light-chain genes of chromosome 2p11 or 22q11 in the other 20%. Burkitt-cell leukaemia is frequently associated with individuals infected with the human immunodeficiency virus (HIV).

CLL is of B-cell origin in 95% of patients and although cytogenetic abnormalities are found in the majority, there are no particular characteristic patterns.

CML is the most homogenous of the leukaemias, with 95% demonstrating a t(9;22) translocation, creating the *BCR/ABL* fusion gene that codes for a constitutively active tyrosine kinase, necessary for disease progression.

Treatment

The initial treatment of acute leukaemia is aimed at achieving remission using combination chemotherapy, in addition to support with red cell and platelet transfusion and prompt treatment of infection with antibiotics. The exact treatment regimen is dependent on the morphological subtype, the prognostic classification and the age and performance status of the patient. In most cases the treatment lasts 12–36 months. Relapse generally occurs within the first 2 years and patients are re-treated with chemotherapy. Remission is achieved in 50% of cases and 10% of patients achieve cure. A different combination of drugs is used but the intensive approach has a greater risk of infection, complications and death. Allogenic stem cell transplant can be considered for young, fit patients.

CLL only requires treatment if symptoms arise. If necessary, this involves chemotherapy in combination with corticosteroids and rituximab (a monoclonal B-cell antibody). Remission can be achieved but relapse is likely in the majority of patients.

In CML, treatment using a tyrosine kinase inhibitor (imatinib and newer derivatives) has increased the 5-year survival rate for those with the *BCR/ABL* fusion gene to greater than 90%.

Prognosis

The prognosis for leukaemia is dependent on age at diagnosis; the extremely young are most at risk, children have a good prognosis and outcome worsens with increasing age. The leukaemia type, cytogenetic profile and white cell count at diagnosis are important prognostic factors.

Of the acute leukaemias, ALL typically has the best prognosis and is the most responsive to treatment, with more than 80% of patients surviving past 5 years.

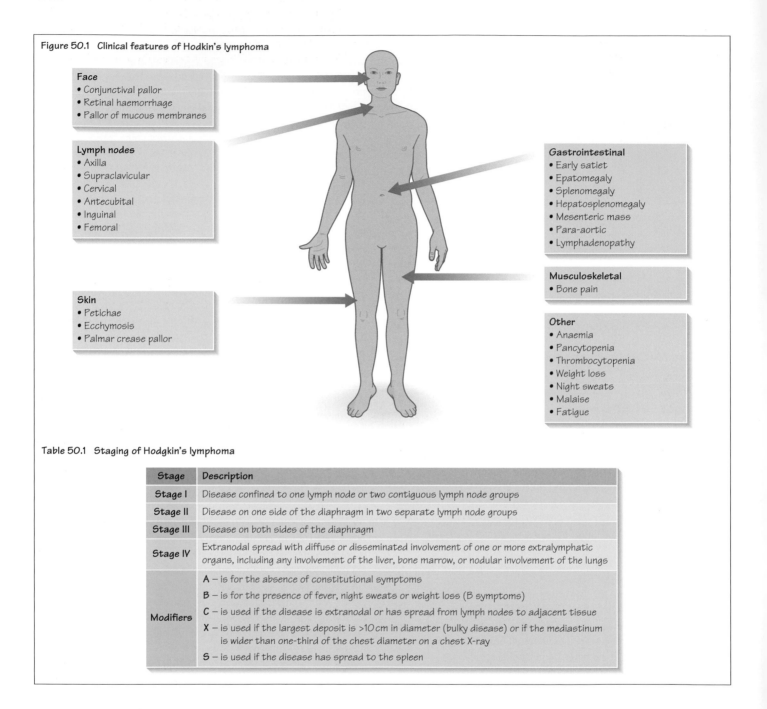

Figure 50.1 Clinical features of Hodkin's lymphoma

Face
- Conjunctival pallor
- Retinal haemorrhage
- Pallor of mucous membranes

Lymph nodes
- Axilla
- Supraclavicular
- Cervical
- Antecubital
- Inguinal
- Femoral

Skin
- Petichae
- Ecchymosis
- Palmar crease pallor

Gastrointestinal
- Early satiet
- Epatomegaly
- Splenomegaly
- Hepatosplenomegaly
- Mesenteric mass
- Para-aortic
- Lymphadenopathy

Musculoskeletal
- Bone pain

Other
- Anaemia
- Pancytopenia
- Thrombocytopenia
- Weight loss
- Night sweats
- Malaise
- Fatigue

Table 50.1 Staging of Hodgkin's lymphoma

Stage	Description
Stage I	Disease confined to one lymph node or two contiguous lymph node groups
Stage II	Disease on one side of the diaphragm in two separate lymph node groups
Stage III	Disease on both sides of the diaphragm
Stage IV	Extranodal spread with diffuse or disseminated involvement of one or more extralymphatic organs, including any involvement of the liver, bone marrow, or nodular involvement of the lungs
Modifiers	A – is for the absence of constitutional symptoms B – is for the presence of fever, night sweats or weight loss (B symptoms) C – is used if the disease is extranodal or has spread from lymph nodes to adjacent tissue X – is used if the largest deposit is >10 cm in diameter (bulky disease) or if the mediastinum is wider than one-third of the chest diameter on a chest X-ray S – is used if the disease has spread to the spleen

Epidemiology

Hodgkin's lymphoma is an uncommon cancer and over the past 50 years advances in radiotherapy and the introduction of combination chemotherapy have tripled the cure rate. Now more than 80% of newly diagnosed patients can expect a disease-free normal lifespan.

More men than women present with Hodgkin's lymphoma and the age-specific incidence of the disease is bimodal, with the greatest peak in the third and seventh decades. The age-specific incidence of Hodg-kin's lymphoma differs markedly in different countries. In Japan, the overall incidence is low and the early peak is absent. In some developing countries, there is a downward shift of the first peak into childhood.

Aetiology

The cause of Hodgkin's lymphoma remains unknown, and there are no well-defined risk factors for its development. However, certain associations have been noted that provide clues to possible aetiological factors. Same-sex siblings of patients with Hodgkin's lymphoma have a 10-fold higher risk for the disease and a monozygotic twin sibling of a patient with Hodgkin's lymphoma has a 99-fold higher risk of developing the disease than a dizygotic twin.

Familial aggregation may imply genetic factors, but other epidemiologic findings mentioned above suggest an abnormal response to an infective agent. The Epstein–Barr virus (EBV) has been implicated by both epidemiological and serological studies in addition to demonstrating the EBV genome in 20–80% of Reed–Sternberg cells. In patients with HIV infection there is a sixfold increase in Hodgkin's lymphoma.

Pathophysiology

Nodular sclerosing (60%) is the most common subtype, typically seen in young adults (more common in females) who have early-stage supradiaphragmatic presentations. It is composed of large tumour nodules, with scattered lacunar classical Reed–Sternberg cells set in a background of reactive lymphocytes, eosinophils and plasma cells with varying degrees of collagen fibrosis/sclerosis. These patients have a good prognosis.

Mixed cellularity (30%) is the second most common histology. It is more common in males, who present with generalised lymphadenopathy or extranodal disease and with associated B symptoms. Reed–Sternberg cells are frequently seen but bands of collagen are absent, although a fine reticular fibrosis may be present. The cellular background includes lymphocytes, eosinophils, neutrophils and histiocytes.

Lymphocyte-predominant (5%) is an infrequent form of Hodgkin's lymphoma, which has the best prognosis. The cellular background is primarily lymphocytes in a nodular or sometimes diffuse pattern. This type may cause diagnostic confusion with nodular lymphocyte-predominant B-cell non-Hodgkin's lymphoma (NHL). This form is often clinically localised and effectively treated with irradiation alone, but may relapse late (reminiscent of low-grade NHL).

Lymphocyte-depleted (5%) is a rare subtype, with large numbers of Reed–Sternberg cells with only a few reactive lymphocytes, diffuse fibrosis and necrosis. This subtype may be associated with HIV infection and is most commonly diagnosed in the elderly. Patients usually have advanced-stage disease, extranodal involvement, an aggressive clinical course and a worse prognosis than with other subtypes.

Clinical presentation

Hodgkin's lymphoma is a lymph node-based malignancy and commonly presents with asymptomatic lymphadenopathy. More than 80% of patients present with lymphadenopathy above the diaphragm, often in the anterior mediastinum, cervical, supraclavicular and axillary regions. Fewer than 20% of patients have involved lymph nodes below the diaphragm, usually in the inguinal region. Disseminated lymph node enlargement is unusual, as is involvement of Waldeyer's ring, occipital, epitrochlear, posterior mediastinal and mesenteric sites.

About 40% of patients have systemic symptoms that include fever, night sweats, weight loss (B symptoms) and chronic pruritus (Table 50.1). These symptoms are more frequent in older patients and have a negative impact on prognosis. Extranodal involvement can be by direct invasion (E lesion) or by haematogenous dissemination (stage IV disease). The most common extranodal sites to be involved are the spleen, lungs, liver and bone marrow.

Investigations and staging

All patients require a careful history and clinical examination. Laboratory studies should include a full blood count, ESR, serum biochemistry for liver and renal function, alkaline phosphatase and LDH. Abnormalities of liver function should prompt further evaluation with imaging and possible biopsy. An elevated alkaline phosphatase is nonspecific but it may indicate bone involvement, which should be evaluated with a bone scan and plain film imaging. A significantly elevated LDH is associated with worse prognosis.

Biopsy of an enlarged lymph node is vital for diagnosis and this should be an excision biopsy as an FNA would be inadequate.

Imaging should include a chest X-ray and CT or MRI of the chest, abdomen and pelvis; however, there is an error rate of 60% in identifying involvement of the liver and spleen. PET imaging can be used to determine the extent of spread and for staging.

Bone marrow involvement is relatively uncommon, but because of the impact of a positive biopsy on further staging and treatment, bone marrow aspirate and trephine should be considered. Staging laparotomy has long been abandoned.

Treatment

Patients with stage I–IIA Hodgkin's lymphoma are generally treated with radiotherapy, unless there are constitutional symptoms or bulky disease. For stage IIB–IV disease, patients require chemotherapy.

Radiotherapy is given to lymphadenopathy above the diaphragm using mantle radiation, which includes the neck, axillae and chest lymph node regions. Below the diaphragm it is administered in an inverted Y field that includes the para-aortic and iliac regions.

Combination chemotherapy uses ABVD (adriamycin, bleomycin, vinblastine and dacarbazine) and studies have shown equivalence to MOPP and other hybrid regimens. Among patients with advanced disease, 70–90% will have a complete response to treatment but up to 35% of patients with stage III–IV disease will relapse, usually within 3 years after treatment.

High-dose chemotherapy followed by stem cell transplantation is the most effective treatment for patients who do not respond to standard-dose chemotherapy. No standard conditioning regimen has been used in this setting, as patients have had prior treatment with a variety of combinations of chemotherapy and radiation therapy. Although most patients who have high-dose treatment have been treated with several regimens or have had less responsive disease from initial diagnosis, the complete response rate is 50–80%, with 40–80% of patients achieving durable remission.

Prognosis

Approximately 90% of patients with small-volume, early-stage disease are cured with radiotherapy and 40–60% of patients with advanced disease are curable with chemotherapy.

Poor prognostic factors for response to first-line chemotherapy include B symptoms, age over 45 years, bulky mediastinal disease, extranodal involvement, low haematocrit, high ESR, and high levels of CD30 and soluble interleukin-2 receptor. Once patients have relapsed, they are classified into three groups: those who achieve a complete response lasting more than 12 months, those who relapse within 12 months and those who never obtain a complete response to first-line chemotherapy.

51 Non-Hodgkin's lymphoma

Figure 51.1 Clinical features of Non-Hodgkin's lymphoma

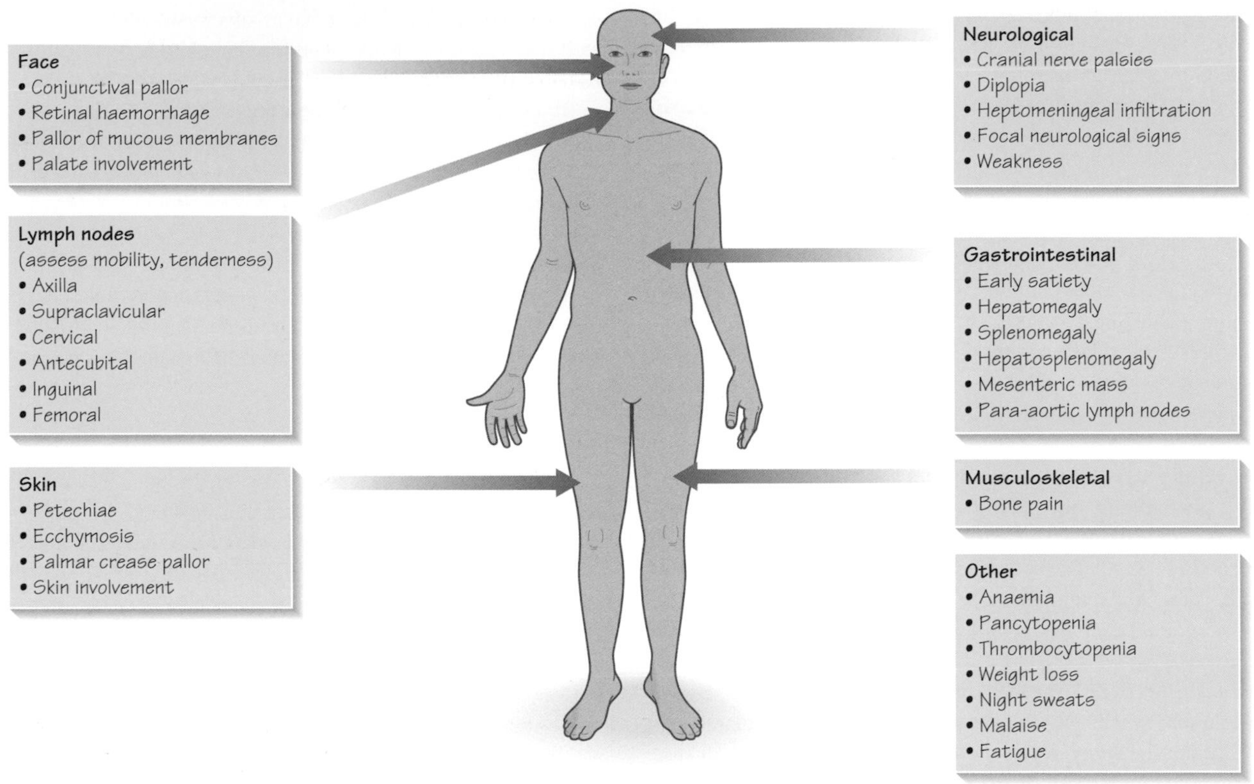
Face
• Conjunctival pallor
• Retinal haemorrhage
• Pallor of mucous membranes
• Palate involvement
Lymph nodes
(assess mobility, tenderness)
• Axilla
• Supraclavicular
• Cervical
• Antecubital
• Inguinal
• Femoral
Skin
• Petechiae
• Ecchymosis
• Palmar crease pallor
• Skin involvement
Neurological
• Cranial nerve palsies
• Diplopia
• Heptomeningeal infiltration
• Focal neurological signs
• Weakness
Gastrointestinal
• Early satiety
• Hepatomegaly
• Splenomegaly
• Hepatosplenomegaly
• Mesenteric mass
• Para-aortic lymph nodes
Musculoskeletal
• Bone pain
Other
• Anaemia
• Pancytopenia
• Thrombocytopenia
• Weight loss
• Night sweats
• Malaise
• Fatigue

Table 51.1 Staging of Non-Hodgkin's lymphoma

Stage	Description
Stage I	Disease confined to one lymph node or two contiguous lymph node groups
Stage II	Disease on one side of the diaphragm in two separate lymph node groups
Stage III	Disease on both sides of the diaphragm
Stage IV	Extranodal spread with diffuse or disseminated involvement of one or more extralymphatic organs, including any involvement of the liver, bone marrow, or nodular involvement of the lungs

Epidemiology

Non-Hodgkin's lymphoma (NHL) is relatively common, with 7500 cases per year in the UK. It is slightly more common in men than women and the median age at presentation for all subtypes of NHL is over 50 years. High-grade lymphoblastic and small non-cleaved-cell lymphomas are the most common types of NHL seen in children and young adults. Low-grade lymphomas account for 37% of cases in patients between the ages of 35 and 64 years at diagnosis but for only 16% of cases in those below the age of 35.

Certain endemic geographical factors appear to influence the development of NHL in specific areas. Human T-cell lymphotrophic virus-1 (HTLV-1)-associated T-cell lymphoma/leukaemia occurs more frequently in Japan (Kyushu) and the Caribbean. Burkitt's lymphoma is more common in Africa, particularly Nigeria and Tanzania. Follicular lymphomas are more common in North America and Europe but are rare in the Caribbean, Africa, China, Japan and the Middle East. Peripheral T-cell lymphomas are more common in Europe and China than in North America. Primary CNS lymphoma is rare, but a significantly higher incidence is seen in patients with HIV infection and immunosuppression.

Aetiology

Non-random chromosomal and molecular rearrangements are important in the pathogenesis of NHL and correlate with histology and immunophenotype. The most commonly associated finding is the t(14;18)(q32;q21) translocation (85% of follicular lymphomas, 28% of high grade tumours), which produces a juxtaposition of the *BCL2* apoptotic inhibitor oncogene to the heavy-chain region of the immunoglobulin locus. The t(11;14)(q13;q32) translocation results in over-expression of *BCL1* (cyclin D1/*PRAD1*), a cell-cycle control gene on chromosome 11q13, and is highly associated with mantle cell lymphoma. Chromosomal translocations involving 8q24 lead to c-myc deregulation and are frequently seen in high-grade small non-cleaved-cell lymphomas (Burkitt's and non-Burkitt's types), including those associated with HIV infection.

Several viruses have been implicated in the pathogenesis of NHL, including EBV (Burkitt's lymphoma), HTLV-1 (adult T-cell leukaemia/lymphoma), human herpesvirus 8 (Kaposi's sarcoma) and HCV (predisposes B-cells to malignant transformation by enhancing signal transduction on binding to the CD81).

Clinical presentation

Patients can present with fever, weight loss and night sweats, referred to as systemic B symptoms, fatigue and weakness (see Chapter 50). These are more common in intermediate- and high-grade tumours but may be present in all stages and tumour subtypes.

Low-grade NHL can present with painless, slowly progressive peripheral lymphadenopathy, which sometimes waxes and wanes. Spontaneous regression of enlarged lymph nodes can occur and can cause a low-grade lymphoma to be confused with an infectious condition. Primary extranodal involvement and B symptoms are uncommon at presentation; however, both are common in advanced or end-stage disease. Bone marrow is frequently involved, sometimes in association with pancytopenia. Splenomegaly is seen in about 40% of patients, but is rarely the only involved site at presentation.

Intermediate- and high-grade lymphomas can present in a more varied manner, with the majority of patients having lymphadenopathy. In 40% of cases this is associated with extranodal involvement, the most common sites being the GI tract (stomach and small intestine), skin, bone marrow, sinuses, oral cavity, GU tract, thyroid and CNS. B symptoms occur in about 40% of patients.

Lymphoblastic lymphoma often presents with an anterior superior mediastinal mass, SVC obstruction and leptomeningeal disease with cranial nerve palsies. Patients with Burkitt's lymphoma present with a large abdominal mass and symptoms of bowel obstruction.

Investigations and staging

Patients require a careful history and clinical examination. Histological evaluation is required with an excision biopsy of an affected lymph node, bone marrow aspiration and trephine. Imaging typically consists of chest X-ray (mediastinal or hilar adenopathy, pleural effusions, parenchymal lesions), and CT of chest and abdomen (mediastinal, hilar, or parenchymal pulmonary disease; para-aortic or mesenteric lymph nodes; splenomegaly; filling defects in liver and spleen). Bone scan is indicated if there are musculoskeletal symptoms or an elevated

alkaline phosphatise. PET imaging is widely used to determine the stage and extent of disease involvement.

Full blood count with differential, serum biochemistry, LDH and β2-microglobulin are required. HIV serology should be considered in patients with diffuse large-cell, immunoblastic and small non-cleaved-cell histology; HTLV-1 serology in patients with cutaneous T-cell lymphoma, particularly if they have hypercalcaemia. Cytogenetic and molecular analyses of lymph node, bone marrow and peripheral blood should be considered. Examination of CSF is required in patients with: diffuse aggressive NHL with bone marrow, epidural, testicular, paranasal sinus, or nasopharyngeal involvement; high-grade lymphoblastic lymphoma and small non-cleaved-cell lymphomas (Burkitt's and non-Burkitt's types); HIV-related lymphoma; and primary CNS lymphoma.

Treatment

Low-grade tumours are frequently disseminated at diagnosis but if they are stage I with small-volume disease, radiotherapy is used. For patients with stage II–IV, systemic treatment is used with oral chlorambucil or intravenous cyclophosphamide, vincristine and prednisolone. Both treatments are associated with bone marrow suppression and can result in neutropenic sepsis.

Rituximab is a monoclonal antibody that targets the CD20 antigen found on the surface of more than 90% of B-cell lymphomas. This is used as a single agent in the treatment of relapsed low-grade NHL and considered in combination with chemotherapy for follicular, mantle cell and diffuse aggressive NHL. When administered weekly for 4–8 weeks, rituximab produces a 60% overall response rate in patients with relapsed low-grade lymphoma.

High-grade and intermediate-grade tumours are more likely to be confined to one lymph node group (stage I) than low-grade tumours and are therefore considered for radiotherapy, although combination chemotherapy with involved field radiotherapy improves outcome. Patients with large-volume stage I disease are treated with chemotherapy using the CHOP regimen. Patients with poor prognosis lymphoma at presentation or at relapse may be considered for high-dose chemotherapy with autologous or allogeneic stem cell transplantation. Long-term immunosuppression is required for patients receiving an allogeneic transplant. There is a treatment-associated mortality of this approach, which may exceed 10%.

Lymphoblastic lymphomas have a propensity for CNS relapse, therefore prophylaxis with intrathecal chemotherapy is incorporated into a combination chemotherapy regimen using alternating drugs, followed by maintenance therapy for 2–3 years. This produces a complete response rate of up to 80% with long-term survival rate of 45%.

Prognosis

Patients with disseminated low-grade tumours are not cured with treatment and although 85% of patients achieve a complete remission, this is transient. Relapse occurs at a median of 18 months and requires further treatment. Transformation into a high-grade lymphoma occurs at a median of 7.5 years after diagnosis.

Patients with low-volume stage I high-grade tumours have a 95% chance of cure and this is only marginally improved with chemotherapy. For more advanced stages, 70–80% of patients achieve remission, which is sustained in up to 60% of cases. High-grade lymphomas such as mantle cell lymphoma and Burkitt's lymphoma have a worse prognosis.

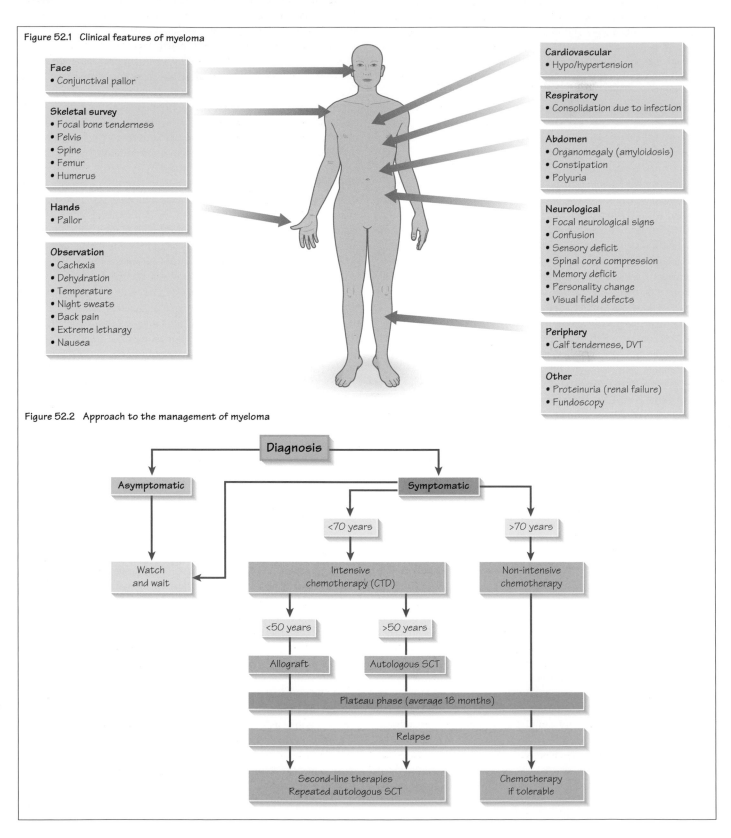

Figure 52.1 Clinical features of myeloma

Face
• Conjunctival pallor

Skeletal survey
• Focal bone tenderness
• Pelvis
• Spine
• Femur
• Humerus

Hands
• Pallor

Observation
• Cachexia
• Dehydration
• Temperature
• Night sweats
• Back pain
• Extreme lethargy
• Nausea

Cardiovascular
• Hypo/hypertension

Respiratory
• Consolidation due to infection

Abdomen
• Organomegaly (amyloidosis)
• Constipation
• Polyuria

Neurological
• Focal neurological signs
• Confusion
• Sensory deficit
• Spinal cord compression
• Memory deficit
• Personality change
• Visual field defects

Periphery
• Calf tenderness, DVT

Other
• Proteinuria (renal failure)
• Fundoscopy

Figure 52.2 Approach to the management of myeloma

Diagnosis

Asymptomatic → Watch and wait

Symptomatic
- <70 years → Intensive chemotherapy (CTD)
  - <50 years → Allograft
  - >50 years → Autologous SCT
- >70 years → Non-intensive chemotherapy

Plateau phase (average 18 months)

Relapse

Second-line therapies
Repeated autologous SCT

Chemotherapy
if tolerable

Epidemiology

Myeloma is a haematological cancer, affecting 4 per 1000 people in the UK population. There is an equal sex distribution, increasing incidence with age and the prevalence is higher in Afro-Caribbean populations. Age is the principal risk factor and most cases present in patients aged 65 years and over. Myeloma rarely occurs in patients under 35 years of age.

Aetiology

Myeloma is a B-cell cancer caused by a clonal proliferation of mature plasma cells that secrete immunoglobulins or fragments thereof. Karyotype abnormalities have been found in 50% of myeloma patients with several molecular events recognised (e.g. 14q32 translocations, chromosome 13 deletions, FGFR3 activation). The clonal population of plasma cells has already undergone immunoglobulin class switching and somatic hypermutation, leading to the overproduction of a single immunoglobulin class, referred to as a paraprotein. Once the plasma cells have mutated they typically migrate to the bone marrow, causing bone marrow infiltration. Dysregulation of the osteoprotegrin rankl system by tumour-secreted cytokines can lead to osteolysis and produce destructive bone lesions.

Clinical presentation

Myeloma frequently presents with significant bone pain due to destructive lytic lesions or pathological fractures that are characteristic of this cancer. Vertebral collapse is common and can lead to spinal cord compression resulting in a precipitous presentation to an emergency department. Otherwise myeloma may present with vague symptoms such as general malaise due to anaemia, ache, discomfort and a history of repeated infections. Increasingly, myeloma is diagnosed due to an incidental finding on a blood count with pancytopenia or anaemia. Important red flags are the presence of unexplained back pain, night sweats, weight loss and extreme lethargy. Complications such as renal impairment and progressive renal failure due to amyloidosis or the deposition of paraprotein in the kidneys may occur. Patients can also develop atypical infections due to pancytopenia.

Investigations and staging

Patients require a full blood count, measurement of ESR and serum protein electrophoresis. In 60% of patients the full blood count will show a normocytic, normochromic anaemia of chronic disease and can demonstrate anaemia or pancytopenia due to marrow infiltration. ESR is raised and serum and urine electrophoresis for immunoglobulins will demonstrate a monoclonal paraprotein band. In some forms of myeloma, paraprotein may only appear in the urine in the form of **Bence Jones protein**. Serum biochemistry should investigate renal function, β2 microglobulin levels and alkaline phosphatase levels; a raised alkaline phosphatase level may indicate bone involvement. Hypercalcaemia is common and needs exclusion. Examination of the peripheral blood film may show the formation of rouleaux and are associated with a very high ESR.

Patients should be referred to a haematologist for further investigation, which will include a bone marrow aspirate and trephine, on which there is typically more than 20% plasma cells seen. These cells are strongly positive for CD138 and cytoplasmic immunoglobulin (cIg) and are negative for CD5, CD20 and surface immunoglobulin (sIg) expression. Normal plasma cells express CD19 but malignant plasma cells in myeloma lose this feature and are CD19 negative, possibly related to loss of *PAX5* gene expression. CD10 expression is generally negative but has sometimes been noted in advanced disease. Monoclonality may be demonstrated by immunoperoxidase staining with κ and λ antibodies and cytogenetic analysis may be helpful.

Plain film X-rays of any sites of bone tenderness should be arranged and can be used to direct subsequent radiotherapy. A skeletal survey is required to assess the extent of bone disease as bone scans are not helpful for detection because they demonstrate osteoblastic activity. Myeloma stimulates osteoclastic activity and is therefore not seen on a bone scan, but hotspots are usually the result of pathological fractures.

Treatment

Initial treatment should be directed at correction of renal function abnormalities and hypercalcaemia. The patient should be started on allopurinol and may require hydration and transfusion. If there is significant bone pain, opiates and radiotherapy may be required.

Treatment is aimed at achieving a remission referred to as plateau phase (Figure 52.2). The myeloma is likely to recur and therefore watchful waiting is adopted for surveillance after treatment, because until symptoms occur, there is no benefit from early intervention.

Direct treatment usually takes the form of chemotherapy, typically a combination of cyclophosphamide, thalidomide and dexamethasone (CTD). This is used to achieve complete remission of the myeloma. Thalidomide can cause teratogenic effects and the patient must be informed of these. It can also cause constipation, peripheral neuropathy and an increased thrombotic risk.

If complete remission is obtained patients may be considered for autologous stem cell transplantation (SCT) as it can prolong the disease-free interval, although unfortunately it does have a high relapse rate. Allogenic stem cell transplantation is considered for more resistant cases and usage must be carefully weighed against risk to the patient.

Supportive therapies include: radiotherapy to treat localised lytic lesions, bone pain and spinal cord compression; blood transfusions for anaemia; and immunisations to protect against common pathogens. Early intervention for bone disease can prevent fractures and the use of bisphosphonates and percutaneous vertebroplasty are important for preserving the axial skeleton.

More recent developments have seen the development of proteasome inhibitors such as bortezomib, which modulates the activity of NF-kappaB, and thalidomide derivatives, such as lenolidamide.

Prognosis

Myeloma is currently not a curable disease. In all cases, it will inevitably reoccur and become increasingly more resistant to therapeutic options, with second- and third-line therapies conferring more risk to the patient. It is important to assess the palliative requirements of the patient and maintain a patient-centred approach to the choice of therapies. The average 5-year survival rate is 35%.

Figure 53.1 Percentage of cases by tumour type and age group

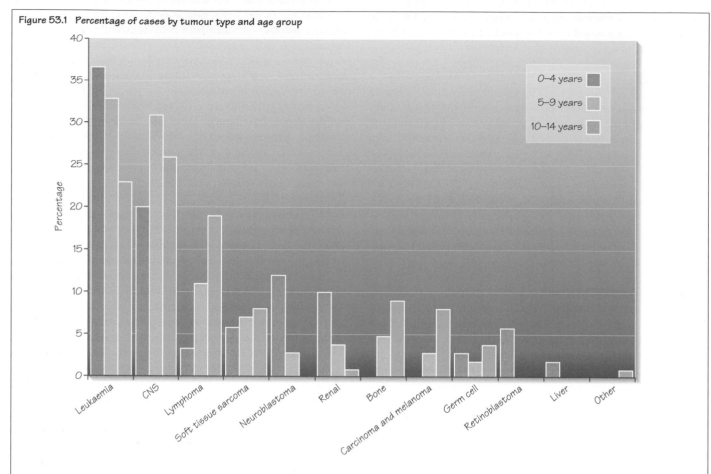

Table 53.1 Distribution of childhood cancers by gender

Cancer	Percentage (%)	Male (%)	Female (%)
Leukaemia	31	55	45
Central nervous system	25	55	45
Lymphoma	10	66	34
Soft tissue sarcoma	7	55	45
Neuroendocrine	6	51	49
Renal cancer	6	46	54
Bone cancer and sarcoma	4	52	48
Carcinoma and melanoma	3	39	61
Germ cell tumours	3	45	55
Retinoblastoma	3	49	51
Hepatic cancer	1	61	39
Other and unspecified cancer	1	50	50

Paediatric oncology

The treatment of children with cancer requires the same general principles of approach to diagnosis, treatment and management as those utilised in adult oncology. However, many of the tumours respond more favourably to chemotherapy than adult cancers do and the goal of treatment is always survival. Chemotherapy and radiotherapy can have devastating long-term consequences in children; increasing their risk of further cancers in later life and limiting bone growth and intellect due to exposure of growing bone and developing brain to radiation. Such issues require careful explanation and consideration when planning treatment in patients of young age.

There are practical considerations when dealing with children, as they are generally not good historians and reliance is placed on the vigilance of parents and carers, which can result in a delayed presentation and hinder the progress of treatment. Children are often scared of hospitals, doctors and medical procedures, so painful procedures such as lumbar puncture or bone marrow aspirates are often carried out under general anaesthetic to minimise the distress. Sedation is often required for imaging such as CT or MRI.

The multidisciplinary approach is of great importance as it is not only the medical and psychological wellbeing of the child that must be addressed, but the ripple effect that a diagnosis of childhood cancer has on the whole family.

Teenager and young adult oncology

National standards for cancer services in the UK recognise that teenagers and young adults (TYA) require specific provision of care. More specifically the improvements in outcomes for TYA lag behind those seen in cancer treatment for the very young and very old. This is due to the differing medical and psychological needs of this group, under-representation of TYA in clinical trials, unique aetiologies and the challenge of coping at a time when they are facing difficult physical, emotional and social challenges of adolescence. This group of patients are often subject to late diagnosis and straddle the crossover of children's (generic) and adult (site-specific) cancer services. As a result TYA units have been commissioned to address this shortfall in service provision.

Specific educational goals include smoking cessation, safe sun exposure, breast and testicular examination, healthy eating and drinking, advice regarding HPV infection and a general promotion of self-awareness of their own health.

Referral pathways are agreed in all cancer networks in the UK, where a primary treatment centre can provide a full range of sustainable services by appropriately trained staff. All care must be provided in age-appropriate facilities and patients must have unhindered access to facilities and support.

Age-appropriate care provides access to cancer expertise that is relevant to young people, where staff work with young people throughout the whole pathway, from bench to bedside. There should be access to peers, with at least some of their treatment happening with patients of a similar age. The care needs to be delivered in an environment that is sensitive to the needs of young people.

Patients aged 19 and over who decide to receive all of their treatment in local adult services should have an individualised treatment plan agreed by the local site-specific MDT and the TYA MDT at the designated primary treatment centre.

Aetiology

Childhood cancers are rare in the UK, with 1500 children diagnosed with cancer each year, representing only 0.5% of all cancers. Cancer still represents the second leading cause of death in children after accidental injury. The incidence of cancer under age 15 years is approximately 140 cases per million children, giving a 1 in 500 risk of developing cancer in childhood. Childhood cancer survival has improved for all types of tumour over the past 50 years, and almost eight out of every 10 children (78%) diagnosed with cancer now survive for 5 years or more.

The types, prevalence and categorisation of cancers affecting children vary noticeably from those seen in adults. Childhood cancers are classified by histology to identify their tissue of origin, rather than by primary tumour site. Table 53.1 outlines the common childhood cancers and their overall prevalence and demonstrates a difference in the prevalence of tumour type by sex; overall, boys are slightly more likely to develop cancer than girls by a ratio of approximately 6:5. The distribution of cancer in children also varies with age, as shown by Figure 53.1.

Haematological cancers

Leukaemia

Leukaemia accounts for almost a third of all childhood cancers and is predominantly acute leukaemia (ALL, 79%; AML, 15%). Acute lymphoblastic leukaemia (ALL) shows a peak incidence at around 2–3 years of age, while acute myeloid leukaemia (AML) is most common in infancy. Presentation is similar to that in adults, with common symptoms of general malaise, easy bruising, bleeding, fever, bone or muscular pain, headache, irritability, shortness of breath and increased incidence of infections. Diagnosis is made on FBC, blood film and bone marrow aspiration. Staging requires imaging and lumbar puncture (see Chapter 49).

Treatment requires intensive combination chemotherapy for all forms of acute leukaemia. Girls with ALL typically receive treatment for 2 years, while boys need 3 years of treatment as their risk of relapse is higher. The 5-year survival for ALL is 88% and AML 64%.

Lymphoma

These cancers are categorised into Hodgkin's lymphoma and non-Hodgkin's lymphoma (NHL). Hodgkin's lymphoma constitutes about two-fifths of all childhood lymphoma and NHL can be subdivided into three main types in children: lymphoblastic, small non-cleaved-cell (Burkitt's lymphoma) and large-cell lymphoma.

In children, the prevalence in boys is twice that of girls and the incidence increases with age (Figure 53.1). Children tend to present with painless swollen lymph nodes noticed as a lump, or by compression of structures such as the airways or bowel, presenting with breathlessness, persistent cough or bowel obstruction. Systemic features include fever, weight loss, diminished appetite, hepatosplenomegaly and night sweats. Diagnosis requires an excision biopsy of an affected lymph node, with bone marrow aspirate and trephine and CT imaging to determine the extent of disease and stage.

Treatment of Hodgkin's lymphoma requires radiotherapy for localised disease, but combination chemotherapy possibly followed by radiotherapy in more advanced disease. Systemic chemotherapy is required for NHL but the requirement for radiotherapy is less.

Overall 5-year survival is very good with 95% for Hodgkin's lymphoma and 83% for NHL (see Chapters 50 and 51).

Embryonal tumours

Embryonal tumours are almost exclusive to childhood, with a peak incidence in the early years of life, and can occur in various tissue types and organs throughout the body. They consist of highly proliferative tissue that is usually only found in the developing embryo. There are four primary types of embryonal tumour.

Neuroblastoma

Neuroblastoma is the most common solid tumour of infancy. The majority of cases are seen in children under 5 years of age and it is almost exclusive to children under 10 years. Tumours often have amplification of the N-myc oncogene and can arise from any site along the craniospinal axis, derived from the neural crest cells that give rise to the sympathetic nervous system. The most common sites are adrenal medulla (35%), pelvis (25%), thorax (15%), and head and neck (5%). As the majority of tumours occur in the abdomen it is typical for a child to present with a large, firm abdominal mass that crosses the midline. Symptoms vary with tumour site and can include breathlessness, dysphagia, weight loss, failure to thrive, fever, pallor, bone metastases (particularly skull) and occasionally a rash of blue coloured bumps where neuroblastoma has infiltrated the skin. Diagnosis is based on CT imaging, blood, bone marrow and urine tests, with approximately 90% of patients having raised levels of vanillylmandelic acid or homovanillic acid in their urine. This can be used for diagnosis and to monitor treatment response. At presentation more than 50% of children will have metastatic disease.

Neuroblastoma is classified as low, intermediate or high risk and treatment is stratified accordingly. In low-risk disease, which has not spread, complete cure may be achieved with surgical resection, while intermediate disease requires chemotherapy after surgery. High-risk disease is very difficult to treat and to maintain remission and requires multimodal therapy with surgery, intensive chemotherapy with stem cell rescue, radiotherapy and immunotherapy using monoclonal antibodies. Overall 5-year survival in neuroblastoma is 55%.

Retinoblastoma

Retinoblastoma is a tumour of the retina of the eye, which results from an inherited fault in the *RB1* gene on chromosome 13 or is due to a sporadic mutation within the gene. A family history of retinoblastoma is strongly suggestive of a heritable form of the disease; however, children with sporadic disease can have a heritable form if the genetic mutation occurred early in embryological development. Heritable *RB1* gene mutations greatly increase the risk of developing bilateral retinoblastoma and of developing other cancers later in life (see Chapter 8). Genetic counselling and screening is offered in all cases of retinoblastoma.

Retinoblastoma is commonly detected due to leukocoria, where an abnormal white light reflex is observed on shining a light in the eye, rather than the expected red light reflex. This may be detected in neonates and infants when performing routine screening or noticed by a parent reviewing a photograph of their child. Less often, the child may develop strabismus or a red, irritated eye, and complain of deteriorating vision, or present with a more general picture of faltering development and growth.

In the UK, survival rates for retinoblastoma are excellent, 99% of children surviving 5 years from diagnosis. The priority of treatment is survival, with the secondary aim to save the child's vision. Treatment approaches include local chemotherapy to the retina and optic nerve, laser therapy, external beam radiotherapy, cryotherapy and surgical removal of the eye.

Nephroblastoma (Wilm's tumour)

This is the most common tumour to affect the genitourinary system of children, accounting for 90% of all renal tumours in children. Most children are fit and healthy prior to developing nephroblastoma but some children with congenital defects such as aniridia, genital and urinary tract abnormalities, and hemihypertrophy are at an increased risk of developing this tumour.

Presentation is often with painless abdominal swelling, with a smooth, firm, non-tender mass, haematuria and occasionally hypertension, malaise or fever. Treatment is surgical resection with adjuvant radiotherapy to the tumour bed in children with a high risk of relapse. Survival has improved greatly, from 59% 30 years ago to 85% more recently.

Hepatoblastoma

Liver tumours are very rare in children and hepatoblastoma accounts for nearly all of them (there are a few cases of hepatocellular carcinoma in older children each year). Children with hepatoblastoma have elevated levels of AFP in their blood, which can be used as a tumour marker to aid diagnosis and to determine response to treatment. It frequently involves the right lobe of the liver and 10% of children have disseminated disease at presentation, with lymph node involvement or lung metastasis.

Surgical resection with or without neoadjuvant chemotherapy has significantly improved the outcome. Small tumours that are surgically resected and treated with adjuvant chemotherapy have a survival that is near 100%. With large tumours, involving most of the liver or with significant residual disease following surgery, liver transplant may be the only remaining option that offers hope.

Central nervous system cancer

In childhood, the brain is the commonest site of solid tumours. Most of these tumours are sporadic, but children with neurofibromatosis, von Hippel–Lindau disease and tuberous sclerosis are at an increased risk and those involved in their care need to be vigilant.

Brain and CNS tumours are graded on their aggressiveness, where grades I and II are low grade, slow growing and generally regarded as benign; grades III and IV are high grade and have malignant potential. These tumours in children have a better outcome than comparable tumours in adults. The two broad groups of malignant brain and CNS tumour in children are glioma and embryonal tumours.

The majority of primary brain tumours in children are benign, but can still cause symptoms when sufficiently enlarged to obstruct CSF flow or result in disruption of normal brain function. Intracranial tumours often produce symptoms due to raised intracranial pressure (ICP), such as nausea and vomiting or headache that is worse on waking. In infants and toddlers, raised ICP may cause lethargy, irritability, poor appetite and result in a general failure to thrive. Cranial nerve palsies can develop and small children can develop macrocephaly. Sensory and motor neurological dysfunction can manifest, but may be very subtle and seizures are possible (see Chapter 47).

Surgical removal of the tumour is the primary goal but if it is invasive, has poorly defined margins or is in an inaccessible area of the brain, complete resection may not be possible. Radiotherapy is used if there is a suspicion of residual disease, but consideration is required to minimise the treatment field in an attempt to limit the damage to normal surrounding brain tissue. Chemotherapy has a clearly defined role in medulloblastoma and is increasingly being used as neoadjuvant treatment to shrink large tumours prior to surgery. Survival is dependent on tumour type and location but overall 5-year survival for CNS tumours is 71%.

Glioma

Gliomas originate in the glial cells of the brain and spinal cord and can be subclassified by their histological resemblance to other cell types. In children, the most common are astrocytomas and ependymomas. Less common types include oligodendroglioma, mixed glioma and choroid plexus tumours. Astrocytomas account for 43% of all childhood CNS tumours and most are intracranial and low grade with 5-year survival of 81%. Ependymomas account for 10% of childhood CNS tumours and arise within the lining of the ventricles, producing symptoms secondary to raised ICP. Their peak incidence is in infancy and 5-year survival is 67%.

Intracranial and intraspinal embryonal tumours

Almost 20% of childhood CNS tumours are embryonal in origin and the most prevalent is medulloblastoma. The incidence is highest in young children and decreases with age. Medulloblastomas most commonly arise in the cerebellum, producing symptoms of raised ICP due to blockage of the ventricles producing hydrocephalus. Patients may complain of headaches over a period of time and have features of papilloedema. MRI imaging of the brain and spinal cord is required. Combinations of surgery, radiotherapy and chemotherapy are required and the 5-year survival is 56%.

Germ cell tumours

Germ cell tumours (GCT) are a diverse group of tumours, broadly categorised into seminomatous and non-seminomatous (NSGCT). They usually occur in the gonads, leading to ovarian or testicular cancer in 43% of cases, but due to the migratory nature of germ cells in the embryo these tumours can occur outside the gonads as the primary site of development. In children, the majority of extragonadal GCTs occur within the CNS, with 34% of all GCTs being either intracranial or intraspinal. The remainder are both extragonadal and extracranial, with sacrococcygeal teratomas a notable example of the commonest tumour found in newborn infants.

When GCTs are gonadal the most common presentation in males is with testicular swelling, most common under 2 years of age and the incidence increases again with the onset of puberty in adolescents. Girls may have a palpable abdominal mass or symptoms of pain or constipation if the tumour invades other abdominal organs. Ovarian GCTs are rare in young girls but the incidence rises with the onset of puberty and continues to increase throughout adolescence (see Chapter 40).

Surgery can be curative if the tumour is localised and easily removed; in such instances chemotherapy can be reserved for salvage treatment in the case of recurrence. These tumours are highly sensitive to chemotherapy, which is required if there is evidence of metastatic spread or complete removal is unlikely. Patients with intracranial GCT require radiotherapy in addition to systemic chemotherapy.

Overall 5-year survival for childhood GCT is 92%.

Soft tissue sarcoma and bone tumours

Sarcomas are a group of tumours that arise in tissues derived from the mesoderm of the embryo, which include bone, muscle, cartilage, fat and vascular tissues. Soft tissue sarcomas can arise throughout the body and the most common type in children is rhabdomyosarcoma, an embryonal tumour of skeletal muscle precursors. This tumour accounts for 53% of childhood sarcomas and is more common in younger children. Rhabdomyosarcoma most commonly occurs in the head and neck, bladder, or testes, and may present as a swelling or lump. Survival in children with this tumour is 63%.

Ewing's sarcoma is a small, round, blue cell tumour, most commonly a tumour of bone, but can occur as a soft tissue tumour and is associated with a t(11;22) chromosomal translocation that juxtaposes *EWS* and *FLI1* genes, resulting in a hybrid transcript. The majority of Ewing's sarcoma of bone arise in the pelvis and the long bones of the limbs, while the majority of soft tissue Ewing's sarcomas arise in the chest.

It is typically a cancer of adolescence and presents with swelling and bone pain, often mistaken for growing pains. Systemic symptoms of fever, weight loss and night sweats may occur. Plain film imaging usually demonstrates ill-defined medullary destruction, periosteal reactions, and new bone formation and soft tissue expansion. Approximately 20% of patients have metastasis at presentation, most commonly involving the lungs or bone (see Chapter 45).

Early detection may allow limb-sparing surgery rather than amputation, but multimodality therapy using surgery, radiotherapy and chemotherapy is standard practice. The 5 year survival is 60%.

Carcinoma and melanoma

Carcinoma is the most common cancer in adults but they are relatively rare in childhood. The incidence of carcinoma and melanoma increases with age in childhood and they are more than twice as likely in 10- to 14-year-olds as they are in the 0- to 4-year-old and the 5- to 9-year-old group combined.

Thyroid cancer most commonly affects adolescent girls who present with painless neck swellings (see Chapter 44).

Malignant melanoma can present as pigmented lesions which show changes in their colour, shape, or size, or demonstrate ulceration or bleeding. Such skin lesions should be treated as suspicious and referred for expert evaluation (see Chapter 46).

Case studies and questions

For each of the following cases, consider the presenting features and collate some ideas about the diagnosis. These cases raise common questions about the condition or scenarios and you should try answering the questions before looking at the answers in the next section.

Case 1: A strong family history of cancer

A 21-year-old woman presented for advice regarding her family history. Her mother was recently diagnosed with breast cancer at the age of 41, her maternal grandmother had ovarian cancer aged 55 and she has two maternal aunts who have both had breast cancer in their 50s.

She is keen to understand her risk and whether she should be referred to a cancer geneticist.
- *What is the likely abnormality?*
- *What is the inheritance and therefore risk that this patient has inherited a mutation from her mother?*
- *What other cancers can be associated with this abnormality?*

Case 2: Fertility preservation after treatment

A 33-year-old woman presented for advice regarding fertility preservation following treatment for a breast cancer. She was married and had been using the oral contraceptive for 10 years and had never been pregnant.

Her planned treatment includes surgery, followed by local radiotherapy and adjuvant systemic chemotherapy with drugs that are likely to induce premature ovarian failure for at least 12 months.
- *What is the likelihood that normal ovarian function will return?*
- *What is the risk of pregnancy on the breast cancer?*
- *What options are available for cryopreservation?*

Case 3: A man with cough and swelling of the face

A 63-year-old man presented with a 2-month history of cough. The family had noted confusion prior to presentation to hospital. He had been complaining of a headache and head fullness, dizziness and visual disturbance. Over the past week his face and neck have become swollen and he had some chest pain. Some of the symptoms were worse when leaning forward, particularly the headache.

On examination there was distension of the cutaneous veins of the upper chest and lower neck, and oedema of the face, neck and arms with some cyanosis of affected areas. Pulse was 80/min and regular, JVP elevated and non-pulsatile. BP and heart sounds were normal, and there was no ankle or sacral oedema. The respiratory rate was 22/min, expansion equal and fair, vocal fremitus normal, percussion dull over left sternal edge, breath sounds diminished in right upper zone with some stridor. Peak expiratory flow rate (PEFR) not done. There was no focal neurological deficit, but mini mental test score was 12/15.
- *What is the most likely complication that has occurred?*
- *What is the most likely cause in this case?*
- *What are the approaches to treatment?*

Case 4: A woman with leg weakness

A 48-year-old woman was receiving chemotherapy for breast cancer and presented with a 2-week history of increasing weakness in the left leg and then right. This was associated with pain in her back and diminished sensation over both legs. The pain was worse on lying flat, weight bearing, sneezing, or coughing.

On clinical examination there was no muscle wasting or fasciculation. There was bilateral leg weakness 3/5 in a pyramidal distribution. Coordination was not assessed. Reflexes were brisk at the knee, ankle and plantars were upgoing. Sensation was diminished in a bilateral and symmetrical distribution up to the level of T11.
- *What is the likely diagnosis?*
- *What is the most likely cause in this case?*
- *What are the approaches to management?*

Case 5: An old man with confusion

A 76-year-old man presented with a 3-month history of cough, occasional haemoptysis and developed a diffuse headache, which was dull and non-throbbing. He had noticed occasional nausea and vomiting and initially attributed this to food. The family noticed a degree of mental confusion, mood and personality changes over the past week. The headache was not worse in the morning and was unaffected by posture or leaning forwards. He was a life-long smoker.

On examination he was dehydrated. There was decreased expansion on both sides of the chest with increased tactile vocal fremitus in the right mid-zone associated with dullness to percussion and bronchial breathing on auscultation. Air entry was fair only in all areas. There was no evidence of organomegaly and no free peritoneal fluid.

There was no evidence of muscle wasting, tone was increased in the right leg, associated with brisk reflexes and an upward plantar response on the right. There was no sensory deficit. Patient was disorientated in time and place, but short- and long-term memory appeared intact. Mini mental test score 9/15.
- *What investigations may be diagnostic?*
- *What are the approaches to management?*
- *What is the most likely underlying cause?*

Case 6: An incidental finding on chest CT

A 45-year-old woman had a recent chest infection and cough. The GP arranged for a chest X-ray as the cough lasted 4 weeks. A nodule was noted and therefore the patient was referred back to her oncologist.

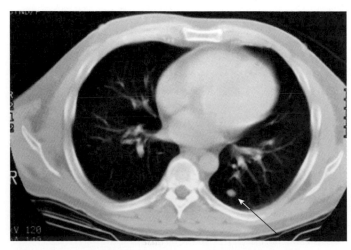

Figure C6.1 A CT of thorax showing a solitary lung nodule in the right lung.

Previously she had a left wide local excision, radiotherapy and chemotherapy for an invasive ductal carcinoma of the left breast, 3 years ago.

On examination there were no peripheral stigmata of disease. All system examination was normal.

- *What is the approach to management of this condition?*
- *What are the prognostic factors?*

Case 7: A man with right upper quadrant pain

A 53-year-old man presented to his GP with a 3-week history of loss of weight, early satiety and discomfort in the right upper quadrant of the abdomen. He had a past history of a Duke's B colorectal cancer 3 years earlier, treated with hemicolectomy and no adjuvant therapy.

On examination he had lost weight. There were no palpable lymph nodes in any nodal region, and no anaemia. He was possibly mildly icteric. There was tenderness in the right upper quadrant with liver enlargement that measured 19 cm in the mid-clavicular line. There was no other organomegaly and no free peritoneal fluid detected.

- *What is the most likely diagnosis?*
- *What factors correlate with survival?*
- *What are the approaches to management?*

Case 8: A woman with hip pain

A 46-year-old woman presented with a 2-week history of pain in the left hip. She had a fall while gardening and the hip has been painful ever since. She had occasional backache, but not worse recently. Pain was worse on weight bearing, flexion and abduction of the hip.

She had breast cancer 4 years ago treated with a wide local excision and radiotherapy for a 1.8 cm grade 2 invasive ductal carcinoma and she continues on tamoxifen.

On examination there was tenderness over the left hip with reduced flexion and abduction due to pain. There was some tenderness over L2/L3 spine and left lateral ribs (8, 9, 10). There was no other focal tenderness in the axial or peripheral skeleton.

- *What investigations may be helpful in obtaining a diagnosis?*
- *What are the approaches to management?*
- *What are the main goals of management?*

Case 9: A man with breathlessness on exertion

A 59-year-old man presented with a 3-week history of dyspnoea, particularly on exertion. He had an occasional cough over the same time period, which was dry and unproductive. He had a dull chest discomfort as tightness.

On examination there was nicotine staining of the left index and second fingers. There was no peripheral lymphadenopathy. There was no evidence of heart failure, and JVP and heart sounds were normal. On chest examination there was reduced expansion on the right, with decreased tactile vocal fremitus, dullness to percussion and diminished breath sounds. Examination of the left hemithorax was unremarkable. PEFR was 450 L/min. All other examination was unremarkable.

- *What do the clinical signs suggest?*
- *What is the most likely underlying cause?*
- *What is the approach to management?*

Case 10: A young woman with a neck swelling

A 39-year-old woman presented with a 1-month history of painless swelling in her left neck and 10 kg weight loss over the preceding 3 months. An ENT surgeon performed a thorough examination of the nasopharynx, oropharynx and indirect laryngoscopy and found no abnormalities. A thoracic CT scan was reported as showing no abnormalities. She had a left low anterior triangle lymph node biopsy, which demonstrated a poorly differentiated squamous cell carcinoma with keratin pearl formation.

- *What is the likelihood of finding a primary site?*
- *What is the likely site if the same histology was found in an inguinal lymph node?*
- *What investigations should be considered if this was adenocarcinoma instead?*

Case 11: A history of asbestos exposure

A 62-year-old man presented with a pleural effusion and had a history of asbestos exposure. A pleural biopsy demonstrated malignant mesothelioma.

- *From which anatomical structures can this tumour develop?*
- *What is the risk of lung cancer associated with asbestos exposure?*
- *What is the risk of mesothelioma with smoking?*
- *What other tumours apart from mesothelioma are associated with asbestos exposure?*

Case 12: A man with hepatomegaly

A 62-year-old Vietnamese man presented with a 3-month history of abdominal pain and swelling. The pain was in the right upper quadrant of the abdomen and was constant without relief. He reported generalised swelling of his abdomen with flatulence, nausea and constipation. Over the previous 6 weeks he had lost 10 kg in weight and developed anorexia. He emigrated to Britain in the 1980s and had previously been healthy apart from recurrent episodes of malaria while he lived in Asia.

On examination he was emaciated but not jaundiced. He was pyrexial 38°C. There was no peripheral lymphadenopathy. Abdominal examination revealed ascites and a tender, enlarged liver with an irregular edge that extended 10 cm below the costal margin.

The initial investigation results were: Hb 8.7 g/dL, WCC 8.2×10^6/L, Plt 167×10^9/L, ESR 70 mm/h, urea & electrolytes normal, bilirubin 15 µmol/L, aspartate aminotransferase 57 U/L, alkaline phosphatase 1157 U/L, gamma glutamyl transferase 469 U/L, amylase 319 U/L, CXR normal.

- *What is the most likely diagnosis?*
- *What investigations will assist in confirming the diagnosis?*

Case 13: A man with weight loss

A 35-year-old man visited his general practitioner with weight loss, an aching sternum, pelvis and lumbar spine. He complained of abdominal fullness after food. A blood film was reviewed:

- *What does the blood film show?*
- *What is the diagnosis?*
- *What other confirmatory test can be performed?*
- *Why does the patient have abdominal fullness?*
- *How common is bone pain in this condition?*
- *Why might the patient become pancytopenic?*

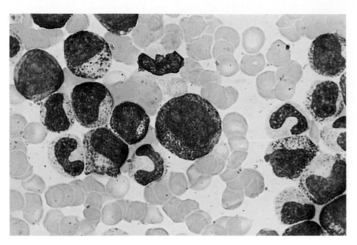

Figure C13.1 Blood film. From Mehta A & Hoffbrand V (2013) *Haematology at a Glance*, 4th edn. Reproduced with permission of Wiley-Blackwell.

Case 14: A woman with an axillary mass

A 45-year-old woman presented with an axillary mass. She had no other complaints, her past medical history was unremarkable and she was not taking any medication.

Clinical examination was unremarkable except for the presence of a firm, non-moveable mass of 4 × 3 cm in the left axilla.

Biopsy of the mass revealed a poorly differentiated malignant cancer without gland formation. Immunohistochemestry of the biopsy was negative for cytokeratin and positive for the leukocyte common antigen.

• *What further investigations would you perform?*
• *What is the most likely diagnosis?*
• *How would you manage this patient if the cytokeritin was positive and the leukocyte common antigen negative?*

Case 15: Confusion and thirst in a smoker

A 65-year-old man was admitted with a large right pleural effusion. He felt thirsty and his family noticed that he had become more muddled. He had a history of significant asbestos exposure 30 years previously. He was a lifelong smoker. On examination, he had clubbing of his fingers.

His blood results showed a serum sodium 131 mmol/L, potassium 3.9 mmol/L, creatinine 72 μmol/L, urea 6.9 mmol/L, corrected calcium 3.10 mmol/L, alkaline phosphatase 100 U/L. A chest X-ray showed a cavitating lesion in the right upper zone.

• *What is the most likely underlying pathology?*
• *What is the cause of the biochemical abnormality?*
• *What steps should be implemented immediately?*

Case 16: Confusion and vomiting

A 70-year-old man presented with confusion, nausea, vomiting and apathy. He was undergoing palliative chemotherapy with carboplatin and etoposide for small cell lung cancer.

His investigations showed serum sodium 119 mmol/L, potassium 2.1 mmol/L, urea 8.9 mmol/L, creatinine 120 μmol/L, corrected calcium 2.12 mmol/L, albumin 30 g/L, aspartate aminotransferase 59 U/L, alkaline phosphatase 247 U/L, gamma glutamyl transferase 260 U/L.

• *What is most likely metabolic disturbance?*
• *What are the criteria to establish a diagnosis?*
• *What is the principal management?*

Case 17: The last hours of life

A 72-year-old woman with end-stage metastatic melanoma was admitted with abdominal pain, shortness of breath and was no longer able to self-care or mobilise. Clinical assessment revealed disease progression and she had previously exhausted all treatment options.

A few days later, the patient was unable to take anything by mouth for several days and was commenced on a subcutaneous infusion of morphine and haloperidol. Despite this she is moaning in discomfort and had myoclonic jerking. All oral medication had been discontinued.

• *What issues would you consider in her management?*
• *What additional medication might improve her symptoms?*

Case 18: Acute problems following chemotherapy

A 28-year-old woman was found to have a stage IV non-Hodgkin lymphoma and started multi-agent chemotherapy. She had no significant medical history. On day 2 of the chemotherapy, she developed a temperature of 39.0°C with rigors and was admitted for investigation.

Her investigations showed a serum sodium of 138 mmol/L, potassium 6.2 mmol/L, creatinine 315 μmol/L, corrected calcium 1.60 mmol/L, phosphate 2.52 mmol/L, lactate dehydrogenase 1238 U/L.

• *What is the most likely cause of the renal impairment?*
• *What additional investigation should be ordered?*
• *What is the approach to immediate treatment?*

Case 19: A woman with facial flushing and diaarhoea

A 58-year-old woman presented with a 6-month history of intermittent facial flushing. Episodes occurred approximately once a week, lasting 15 minutes and were associated with bouts of watery diarrhoea lasting 1 day. She had a long history of well-controlled asthma but recently had become more wheezy, requiring regular inhaler usage.

On clinical examination she was rather plethoric with multiple cutaneous telangiectasia and a rash of small blisters over her neck and hands. There was expiratory wheeze throughout both lung fields with a prominent venous wave in the neck, a third heart sound and a systolic murmur at the left sternal edge, which was louder on inspiration. She had an enlarged liver measuring 6 cm below the costal margin in the mid-clavicular line, which was pulsatile. There was no splenomegally or peripheral lymphadenopathy.

• *What three investigations would you perform?*
• *What cardiac lesion does she have?*
• *What is the cause of her rash?*
• *List two other chronic complications of this condition.*

Case 20: Temperature following chemotherapy

A 32-year-old-woman presented 10 days after a cycle of chemotherapy for Hodgkin's disease. She had developed a temperature and felt hot and cold with one episode of rigor. The chemotherapy information sheet advised her to seek assistance if she developed a temperature, so she presented to casualty.

On examination she was febrile at 38.5°C and looked dehydrated. Her pulse was regular at 100/min, low volume. BP 95/60 mmHg. JVP was not elevated and heart sounds were normal. Chest examination was normal and whe had slight non-specific abdominal tenderness with no organomegaly.

- *What is the most likely cause of this condition?*
- *What are the most important investigations to consider?*
- *What treatment is required?*
- *Are there any preventative measures that can be taken?*

Answers to case studies

Case 1: A strong family history of cancer

- This family is likely to have a mutation in *BRCA1*. This is a germ line mutation that increases the risk of ovarian, breast and colon cancer in females, and prostate and colon cancer in males. *BRCA2* mutations have a greater association with pancreatic cancer and male breast cancer.
- The mutation is inherited as an autosomal dominant pattern with variable penetrance, and if her mother has a mutation, the risk of carrying the gene for this patient is 50%.
- The strong family history warrants referral to a cancer geneticist for testing and consideration of more intensive surveillance.

See Chapter 8.

Case 2: Fertility preservation after treatment

- Treatment for breast cancer cannot be delayed to allow a pregnancy to complete. She should have a discussion relating to prognosis and likely outcome of treatment and effects on fertility and options available for preservation of ovarian function.
- Pregnancy in a woman previously treated for breast cancer does not appear to have an adverse effect on the risk of breast cancer recurrence. Should it recur during a pregnancy there will be issues about whether to treat the cancer during a pregnancy or to terminate.
- There is a high probability that the planned chemotherapy will suppress her ovarian function, but this recovers in at least 70% of patients under 35 years. She could consider fertilised embryo cryopreservation but this would take at least 1 month to complete. This may not be appropriate for a single woman. All other methods should be considered experimental but include storage of mature oocytes and ovarian slice autotransplantation.

See Chapter 29.

Case 3: A man with cough and swelling of the face

- Obstruction of the superior vena cava (SVC) is the clinical expression of obstruction of blood flow through the vessel. Characteristic symptoms and signs may develop quickly or gradually and is caused by compression, invasion, or thrombosis in the superior mediastinum.
- Symptoms and signs may be aggravated by bending forward, stooping, or by lying down.
- Treatment is directed at the underlying cause, and prognosis of patients with SVC obstruction strongly correlates with the prognosis of the underlying disease. Options for treatment include chemotherapy, radiotherapy, endovascular stenting, thrombolysis and surgery. In this case systemic chemotherapy following stenting would be most appropriate.
- In this case, the preceding cough suggests a lung primary and 50% of patients presenting with SVC obstruction have small cell lung cancer.

See Chapter 13.

Case 4: A woman with leg weakness

- The finding of bilateral UMN signs should be considered spinal cord compression until proved otherwise. Spinal cord compression from metastatic cancer remains an important source of morbidity despite the fact that with early diagnosis, treatment is effective in 90% of patients.
- Malignant spinal cord compression is defined as the compressive indentation, displacement, or encasement of the spinal cord's thecal sac by metastatic or locally advanced cancer. Compression can occur via posterior extension of a vertebral body mass, resulting in compression of the anterior aspect of the spinal cord, or through anterior or anterolateral extension of a mass arising from the dorsal elements or invading the vertebral foramen, respectively. Intramedullary spinal cord metastases produce oedema, distortion and compression of the spinal cord parenchyma, resulting in symptoms and signs that are similar to epidural spinal cord compression.
- Any neoplasm capable of metastasis or local invasion can produce malignant spinal cord compression. Response to non-surgical therapy and the duration of survival following treatment can vary considerably among different histologic tumour types. The degree of pre-treatment neurologic dysfunction is the strongest predictor of treatment outcome. Ambulation can be preserved in more than 80% of patients who are ambulatory at presentation. Paraplegia, quadriplegia and loss of bowel or bladder function are potential consequences of cord compression if it is diagnosed late or left untreated, and once lost, neurologic function cannot be regained in the majority of patients.
- The key to successful management is a heightened awareness of signs and symptoms, specifically newly developed back pain or motor dysfunction, leading to early diagnosis and treatment.
- All patients require an urgent MRI and should be discussed with a neurosurgeon, started on dexamethasone and considered for radiotherapy.

See Chapter 13.

Case 5: An old man with confusion

- This patient is likely to have brain metastases, which are a common complication in cancer patients and an increasingly important cause of morbidity and mortality. In adults, metastases are the most common cause of brain tumours, five to 10 times more frequently than primaries. In children, the most common sources are sarcomas, neuroblastoma and germ cell tumours. Certain tumours almost never metastasise to the brain including oesophagus, oropharynx, prostate and non-melanoma skin cancers.
- Brain metastases develop when tumour cells originating in tissues outside the nervous system spread secondarily to directly involve the brain, and develop in 10–30% of adults and 6–10% of children with cancer. The number of cases may be increasing as a result of the increased ability of MRI to detect small metastases.
- Most patients receive effective palliation with systemic chemotherapy and radiotherapy.
- Metastases may involve the brain parenchyma, the cranial nerves, the blood vessels (including the dural sinuses), the dura, the leptomeninges and the inner skull table. Most common are intraparenchymal metastases.
- A CT or MRI (contrast enhanced) may be diagnostic and in some cases a biopsy may be required to exclude a primary tumour.
- Management includes steroids for peritumoural oedema, anticonvulsants, treatment of venous thromboembolic disease (20% of

patients with brain metastases), surgery (single and multiple metastases), whole brain radiotherapy, stereotactic radiotherapy and chemotherapy.

See Chapter 14.

Case 6: An incidental finding on chest CT

• Pulmonary metastases from sarcomas or other distinctive non-pulmonary cancers are usually easy to diagnose, but solitary metastasis from breast or colon, or squamous cell cancer metastasis from head and neck primary tumours, are difficult to distinguish from primary lung cancer.

• Patients with two or more pulmonary nodules can be considered to have metastases.

• A biopsy with comparison of the primary neoplasm and the lung nodule is required; electron microscopy or specific molecular or genetic characteristics may identify more precisely the origin of such cancers; monoclonal antibodies can assist in discriminating between primary bronchogenic adenocarcinoma and colon carcinoma metastatic to the lung; characteristics of amplified K-ras oncogene expression present in the primary tumour can be used to identify pulmonary metastases; flow cytometry and DNA analysis have been used to describe primary carcinomas of the lung and to distinguish them from metastases.

• Prognostic indicators generally associated with prolonged post-resection survival include resectable tumour, longer disease-free interval, longer tumour doubling time, fewer numbers of metastases and solitary metastasis. Neither age nor gender should be considered as prognostic factors.

• The approaches to treatment include surgery with a generous wedge resection, radiotherapy, chemotherapy, endocrine therapy for breast or prostate cancer, and novel therapies.

See Chapter 14.

Case 7: A man with right upper quadrant pain

• Metastatic cancer in the liver can represent the sole or life-limiting component of disease for many patients with a variety of tumour histologies, including colorectal cancer, ocular melanoma, neuroendocrine tumours and occasionally other histologies. The liver is a common site of metastasis for tumours arising in the GI tract.

• Once metastases to the liver are diagnosed, the prognosis is generally poor. Median survival for patients with colorectal cancer in the liver is 12–24 months. In patients with colorectal cancer, the ability to resect disease is associated with 5-year disease-free survival in 20–50% of patients.

• Patients with liver metastases from functional neuroendocrine tumour can derive substantial palliative benefit from resection.

• Synchronous hepatic metastases occur in 10–20% of patients with colorectal cancer. It is the sole or life-limiting component of disease in up to 60% of patients and only a small proportion of patients have resectable disease.

• In colorectal cancer, survival with liver metastasis correlates with extent of disease, number of hepatic nodules, bilobar disease, abnormal liver test results, stage of the primary tumour and number of positive lymph nodes.

• Liver resection can be considered but the mortality associated with major hepatic resection is less than 5%. Death is most commonly secondary to inadequate hepatic synthetic reserve, and complications from hepatic resection include biliary fistula, haemorrhage, abscess, or wound infection.

• Other treatment options include chemoembolisation, local ablative therapy, cryotherapy, cryotherapy plus adjuvant chemotherapy, microwave tissue coagulation and radiofrequency ablation, interstitial laser photocoagulation, percutaneous ethanol injection and whole liver irradiation with or without chemotherapy.

See Chapters 14 and 34.

Case 8: A woman with hip pain

• Most of the people who die of cancer each year have tumour metastasis and bone is the third most common organ involved by metastasis, behind lung and liver. In breast cancer, bone is the second most common site of metastatic spread, and 90% of patients dying of breast cancer have bone metastasis.

• Breast and prostate cancers metastasise to bone most frequently, which reflects the high incidence of both of these tumours, as well as their prolonged clinical courses. Other tumours that commonly cause symptomatic bone metastases include kidney and thyroid cancer, and multiple myeloma.

• Patients with bone metastasis from breast cancer have an average 2-year survival from the time of presentation with their first bone lesion. More patients are living with bone metastases, and thus the challenge is to improve their quality of life.

• Early detection and aggressive management of metastases is the goal to maintain and maximise patients' quality of life and functional level.

• Metastatic bone disease most often presents with pain as the principal symptom. The pain comprises two components: biological and mechanical. Biological pain is related to the local release of cytokines and chemical mediators by the tumour cells, periosteal irritation, stimulation of intraosseous nerves by these mediators, and the pressure or mass effect of the tumour tissue within the bone. Mechanical pain is related to the loss of bone strength and stiffness caused by the metastatic lesion, which leads to activity-related pain, and is seen most often with osteolytic lesions but can also occur in osteoblastic lesions, because the disorganised pattern of tumour-related bone lacks structural integrity.

• Symptoms are intermittent but may be sharp and severe. Pain tends to be worst at night and may be partially relieved by activity. Symptoms become more constant and take on a more mechanical character.

• Patients with metastatic disease can present with a pathological fracture, which occur most often with osteolytic lesions. The majority of pathologic fractures are seen in patients with metastatic breast cancer, with an incidence of 8%, with 53% of those fractures occurring secondary to breast cancer metastases. Other culprits for pathological fracture are kidney 11%, lung 8%, thyroid 5%, lymphoma 5% and prostate 3%.

• There are four main goals in managing patients with metastatic disease to the skeleton: pain relief; preservation and restoration of function; skeletal stabilisation; and local tumour control (e.g. relief of tumour impingement on normal structures, prevention of release of chemical mediators that have local and systemic effects).

• Therapeutic approaches include bisphosphonates, chemotherapy and hormonal therapy, external beam radiotherapy, pain relief, systemic radionuclides and surgery.

See Chapters 14 and 29.

Case 9: A man with breathlessness on exertion

• This man has a pleural effusion and 40% of these are due to malignancy. Cancer is the second leading cause of pleural effusion in patients older than 50 years and it is the initial manifestation in 10–50% of cancer patients.

• The presence of malignant effusion frequently indicates advanced and incurable disease, and the overall prognosis of patients with malignant pleural effusion depends on the histology.

• Accumulation of fluid within the pleural space may be due to: increased hydrostatic pressure in the microvascular circulation; decreased oncotic pressure in the microvascular circulation; decreased pressure in the pleural space; increased permeability of the microvascular circulation; impaired lymphatic drainage from the pleural space; transudation of fluid from the peritoneum via lymphatics; or anatomic defects in the diaphragm.

• Malignant pleural effusions are due to: lung carcinoma (35%), breast carcinoma (23%), lymphoma (10%), carcinomas of unknown primary origin (12%) and other (20%).

• Treatment should focus on palliation of symptoms and be tailored to the patient's physical condition and prognosis; 54% of patients die within 1 month and 84% within 3 months after diagnosis.

• Thoracentesis may be an appropriate treatment for malignant pleural effusion in patients with limited life expectancy who cannot tolerate any surgical procedure, but recurrent effusions are observed in 97% of individuals within 30 days after thoracentesis. Pleurodesis immediately after thoracentesis is not effective, since residual pleural fluid dilutes the sclerosing agent, thus diminishing its irritant effects on the pleura. Loculations may form after such treatment, rendering definitive therapy of the pleural effusion more complicated.

• In patients presenting with malignant pleural effusion as the initial manifestation of breast cancer, small cell lung cancer, germ cell tumours, or lymphoma, thoracentesis followed by systemic chemotherapy may successfully treat disease in the pleural space. Most patients with malignant pleural effusion require more aggressive intervention to prevent recurrence.
See Chapters 14 and 30.

Case 10: A young woman with a neck swelling

• For most patients who present with metastatic disease, routine examination and investigation will quickly disclose the underlying primary tumour. In 1–5% of patients the primary site remains undisclosed because it is too small to be detected or has regressed. The usual histological diagnosis in these patients with unknown primary site is adenocarcinoma or poorly differentiated carcinoma.

• Five highly treatable subsets of unknown primary site have been identified which have more favourable outcomes and require distinct management: breast cancer; primary peritoneal cancer; extragonadal germ cell tumours; neuroendocrine tumours; head and neck tumours.

• The majority of unknown primary tumours do not fit into any of these subsets and the resulting response rates to chemotherapy are <20%, usually of brief duration and have little impact on overall survival. Two-thirds of unknown primary cancer patients have metastatic adenocarcinoma with involvement of two or more visceral sites, usually some combination of liver, lung, lymph nodes and bone

• Investigations for squamous cell carcinoma in cervical nodes include: meticulous inspection of scalp and skin for a primary tumour; ENT examination, indirect laryngoscopy ± examination under anaes-

thesia (EUA) with blind biopsies from nasopharynx and base of tongue; CXR (± thoracic CT); upper GI endoscopy; colposcopy and cervical smear.

• Investigations for squamous cell carcinoma in inguinal nodes include: careful examination of legs, vulva, penis, perineum for primary tumour; pelvic examination (exclude vaginal/cervical cancer); proctoscopy/colposcopy (exclude anal/cervical cancer).

• Investigations for metastatic adenocarcinoma include: oestrogen receptor (ER) and progesterone receptor (PR) expression by the tumour in females; serum PSA in males; serum AFP and hCG (if positive, histology needs review); consider diagnosis of poorly differentiated lymphoma, exclude with immunophenotyping

• In this case the most likely diagnosis is metastatic cervical squamous cell cancer and second most common is squamous oesophageal cancer.
See Chapters 28 and 39.

Case 11: A history of asbestos exposure

• Mesothelioma can arise in the pleura, peritoneum and tunica vaginalis testis, with benign fibrous mesotheliomas described in the atrioventricular node, mediastinum, liver and adrenal gland, arising from mesothelial or submesothelial cells.

• The risk of lung cancer is increased (relative risk of 1.5–13.1). Some studies suggest that asbestos exposure accounts for approximately 5% of lung cancer deaths in men. Relative risk of lung cancer appears to fall following cessation of exposure.

• There is no known direct association of smoking with malignant mesothelioma. However, smoking is synergistic with asbestos exposure and some reports suggest that the risk of developing malignant mesothelioma in patients with asbestos exposure and who smoke is up to 40-fold higher than in those who never smoke.

• Lung cancer is the most common, with a modest increase in gastrointestinal cancers and some suggestion of an increase in other cancers such as those of the kidney, pancreas, oesophagus, colon and larynx.
See Chapter 31.

Case 12: A man with hepatomegaly

• In a patient from Asia presenting with hepatomegaly, fever and liver dysfunction, the most likely diagnosis is hepatocellular carcinoma. This is likely to be associated with a history of hepatitis B or C and appropriate serology should be checked to confirm prior infection.

• Appropriate investigations include CT imaging of the abdomen or ultrasound of the liver and fine needle biopsy of the liver under image-guidance, although this does risk seeding the tumour outside the liver; serum alpha-fetoprotein is raised in 75% of cases.
See Chapter 36.

Case 13: A man with weight loss

• The blood film shows a marked left-shift, with promyelocytes, band forms and neutrophils.

• The diagnosis is chronic myelocytic leukaemia, which can be confirmed with cytogenetic analysis for the Philadelphia chromosome t(9:22).

• Enlargement of the spleen is a common feature and produces abdominal fullness and early satiety.

• Bony aches are common in CML.

• Pancytopenia may be consequent on refractory splenomegaly or rarely due to bone marrow necrosis.
See Chapter 49.

Case 14: A woman with an axillary mass

- Further investigations should include: CT imaging of the thorax, abdomen and pelvis; bone marrow aspirate and trephine; serum β2-microglobulin; and serum immunoglobulins.
- In view of the positive leukocyte common antigen, a non-Hodgkin's lymphoma is the most likely diagnosis.
- In general, women who present with an isolated axillary mass that proves to be adenocarcinoma or poorly differentiated carcinoma should receive treatment appropriate for stage II breast cancer. They should receive either a modified radical mastectomy or breast irradiation for purposes of decreasing local recurrence followed by adjuvant systemic therapy with chemotherapy or tamoxifen or both, depending on menopausal status and the hormone receptor status of the tumour.
- Patients whose routine pathology reveals either poorly differentiated adenocarcinoma or poorly differentiated malignancy deserve a careful pathological review to determine if there are any findings compatible with a specific organ of origin. In this case, the absence of cytokeratin filaments argues against the diagnosis of breast carcinoma; on the other hand, the leukocyte common antigen positivity is highly consistent with a lymphoid tumour. The patient would be expected to respond to therapy as if she had a more straightforward presentation of lymphoma. To determine the optimal therapy for such a patient, the disease should be staged as in any non-Hodgkin's lymphoma. Therefore, CT imaging should be performed to determine whether there are additional sites of disease.

See Chapter 51.

Case 15: Confusion and thirst in a smoker

- Hypercalcaemia is the most common metabolic complication of malignancy. It is particularly common in squamous cell carcinoma, in this case originating in the lung.
- In 80% of cancer-associated cases it is due to parathyroid hormone-related peptide (PTHrP) production by the tumour. PThRP acts on the bone, kidney and gastrointestinal system to increase serum calcium levels. The remaining 20% are due to local resorption of bone by osteoclasts in areas of marrow space with malignant cells.
- The mainstay of treatment is rehydration using large volumes of intravenous fluids followed by a bisphosphonate such as pamidronate. Normalisation of calcium occurs in 80% of patients but may take up to 3 days. In the remaining 20% alternative treatments include somatostatin analogues such as octreotide, calcitonin and mithramycin. Any medication that may elevate calcium, such as thiazide diuretics, should be discontinued.

See Chapter 12.

Case 16: Confusion and vomiting

- Hyponatraemia is common in advanced cancer; however, urine osmolarity assessment is required as the finding of concentrated urine in conjunction with hypo-osmolar plasma suggests abnormal renal free water excretion and the diagnosis of the syndrome of inappropriate antidiuresis (SIAD). Significant symptoms occur when the serum sodium is below 125 mmol/L and can progress to stupor, coma and seizures.
- The essential criteria to establish this diagnosis are:
  - plasma osmolality <275 mosmol/kg H_2O
  - plasma sodium <135 mmol/L
  - urine osmolality >100 mosmol/kg H_2O
  - normal plasma/extracellular fluid volume
  - high urinary sodium (urine sodium >20 mmol/L).

- Supportive criteria for this diagnosis are:
  - abnormal water load test (unable to excrete >90% of a 20mL/kg water load in 4h, and/or failure to dilute urine to osmolality <100 mosmol/kg H_2O)
  - elevated plasma arginine vasopressin levels.
- In euvolaemic hyponatraemia, treatment is with fluid restriction and domeclocycline. Hypertonic saline can be used if the onset of symptoms was rapid or severe. A loop diuretic may help correct hyponatraemia but should be used with caution. Treatment of the underlying cancer may reduce ectopic ADH secretion and improve the patient's symptoms.

See Chapter 12.

Case 17: The last hours of life

- Following assessment of the patient, it is important to spend time with the family to explain the intended management plan. This is an opportunity to outline the expectations of the following hours and discuss the goals of management. The discussion can determine the level of understanding, level of acceptance of the futility of further anticancer therapy and the imminence of the patient's death.
- Moaning is most likely due to pain and discomfort, possibly bone metastasis in this particular case. Faecal impaction and urinary retention should be excluded as possible causes of the discomfort and a careful review of the analgesia dosing is required.
- Myoclonus can be distressing for the patient and their relatives and can be due to the accumulation of opioid metabolites. If there is deteriorating renal function, this may require a reduction in opioid dose or increase in the dosing interval. Benzodiazepines such as midazolam can reduce the myoclonus.
- It is important to prepare the family for the death itself. Continue to explain the management and goals at every opportunity and explain the likely events that may follow.

See Chapter 27.

Case 18: Acute problems following chemotherapy

- The acute destruction of a large number of cancer cells is associated with bulky, chemosensitive disease including lymphoma, leukaemia and germ cell tumours, and can cause tumour lysis syndrome. This results in transient hypocalcaemia, hyperphosphataemia, hypcruricaemia and hyperkalaemia. Patients develop acute renal failure and present with symptoms associated with multiple underlying electrolyte abnormalities, including fatigue, nausea, vomiting, cardiac arrhythmia, heart failure, syncope, tetany, seizures and sudden death.
- Patients should have serum uric acid measured and consider a renal ultrasound in those with pelvic disease to exclude post-renal obstruction.
- Serum biochemistry should be monitored regularly for 48–72 hours after treatment in patients at risk. Good hydration and urine output should be maintained throughout treatment administration. Prophylaxis with allopurinol should be considered and recombinant urate oxidase (rasburicase) can be used to reduce uric acid levels when other treatments fail. Adequate hydration is vital as it has a dilution effect on the extracellular fluid, improving electrolyte imbalance, and increases circulating volume improving filtration in the kidneys. In high-risk patients, hydration should be commenced 24 hours before the start of treatment.

See Chapter 12.

Case 19: A woman with facial flushing and diarrhoea

• She is likely to have carcinoid syndrome due to metastasis from a primary site (most likely in the gastrointestinal tract) to the liver producing hepatomegaly.

• Investigations should include: 24-hour urinary 5-hydroxyindolacetic acid estimation; contrast enhanced CT of the chest and abdomen or somatostatin receptor scintography to localise the tumour and metastases; and two-dimensional echocardiogram with doppler flow studies.

• The clinical signs suggest a complication of tricuspid incompetence secondary to fibrosis of chordae tendini.

• Pellagra can occur due to secondary niacin deficiency on account of niacin usage by the tumour.

• Other complications include arthropathy, pulmonary stenosis, mesenteric fibrosis and cirrhosis.

See Chapter 48.

Case 20: Temperature following chemotherapy

• She is likely to have neutropenic sepsis as an oncological emergency and should be investigated with blood cultures, FBC, chemistry, CXR, urine culture and swab from central line (if present).

• She should be started on high-dose intravenous antibiotics, according to local protocol, which reflects the antibiotic resistance in the local population. First-line empirical therapy is either monotherapy with an antipseudomonal β-lactam (ceftazidime, cefotaxime, or meropenem) or a combination of an aminoglycoside and a broad-spectrum penicillin with antipseudomonal activity (gentamicin + tazocin). Metronidazole may be added if anaerobic infection is suspected. Flucloxicillin or teicoplanin if Gram-positive infection is suspected. Antibiotics should be adjusted according to culture results, although these are often negative. If there is no response after 36–48 hours review antibiotics with microbiologist advice and consider antifungal cover. Her oncologist should be notified immediately to arrange urgent review within 24 hours of admission.

• Colony-stimulating factors are not routinely used for all patients with neutropenia and guidelines for their use have been established. The use of prophylactic antibiotics is considered for some patients at high risk.

• Other supportive therapy that might be required includes intravenous fluids, inotropic support, ventilation and haemofiltration.

See Chapter 13

Glossary

Adjuvant chemotherapy. Treatment administered after a debulking procedure, where the chemotherapy is designed to eradicate the micrometastatic disease that remains. The goal is achieving an improvement in disease-free and overall survival.

Akathisia. Restless legs, associated with an emotional sense of agitation, even in the absence of motor movements.

Aneuploidy. Individual with one or more chromosomes in addition to, or missing from, the complete chromosome set. An example would be trisomy 21 (47XX+21).

Apoptosis. Programmed cell death in which cells take an irreversible step to suicide, resulting in cellular fragmentation and destruction.

Atrophy. A reduction in growth due to a decrease in size or number of constituent parts of a tissue, for example a reduced size of the ovaries following the menopause.

Chemoprevention. The use of pharmacological agents to prevent cancer developing in patients identified at particular risk.

Complete remission. A state where all signs and symptoms of the cancer have disappeared, although cancer still may be in the body.

CT simulation. The patient has a normal CT study and a three-dimensional transformation of the CT image slices is computed and a digitally reconstructed radiograph (DRR) created. The DRR resembles a normal diagnostic film, on which the outlines of the tumour and organs can be drawn by the oncologist to guide radiotherapy treatment.

Cytokeratins. Intermediate filament proteins expressed in pairs as a type I (CK9-20) and type II (CK1-8) on the surface of cells. Different tissues express different patterns of expression and can aid diagnosis on the origins of a particular cell.

Deletion. The loss of a chromosome segment from a normal chromosome.

Disease-free survival. The length of time after treatment for cancer during which a patient survives with no symptoms or signs of the disease. Disease-free survival may be used in a clinical trial to measure how well a new treatment works.

Duplication. An extra piece of chromosome segment that may either be attached to the same or homologous chromosome, or be transposed to another chromosome in the same genome.

Dysplasia. This is an early change that can eventually lead to neoplasia, and the changes do not necessarily revert to normal once the injury stimulus is removed.

Dystonia. A frightening symptom for patients who are receiving metoclopramide, occurring soon after receiving the drug and due to action on dopaminergic receptors. It produces sustained muscle contractions, causing twisting and repetitive movements or abnormal postures.

Electron volt. Photon absorption in human tissue is determined by the energy of the radiation as well as the atomic structure of the tissue in question. The basic unit of energy used is the electron volt (eV); 10^3 eV = 1 keV, 10^6 eV = 1 MeV.

Exposure. In order to measure the dose of radiation received by a patient, the ionisation produced in air by a beam of radiation must be measured. This quantity is known as exposure and the presence of soft tissue can be factored into the calculation of the absorbed dose in Gy.

Gray (Gy). The basic unit of radiation absorbed dose is the amount of energy (joules) absorbed per unit mass (kg), expressed as 1 Gy = 1 Joule/kg tissue. The *gray*, has replaced the obsolete unit of *rad*.

Hyperplasia. An increase in the size of an organ or tissue due to an increase in the number of cells, for example a lactating breast.

Hypertrophy. An increase in the size of an organ or tissue due to an increase in the size of individual cells, for example cardiomegaly resulting from increased cardiovascular strain.

Inflammatory pain. The result of peripheral or central mediators of inflammation that can create feedback loops which sensitise primary afferent nerves causing peripheral hyperalgesia. These can be inhibited peripherally via opioid receptors or COX pathways.

Invasion. The ability to infiltrate the surrounding tissues and organs, which is a characteristic of malignancy.

Inversion. A change in linear sequence of the genes in a chromosome that results in the reverse order of genes in a chromosome segment. Inversions can be pericentric with two breaks on either side of the centromere, or paracentric with both breaks on the same arm.

Isochromosome. Breaks in one arm of a chromosome followed by duplication of the other arm of the chromosome to produce a chromosome with two arms that are both short (p) or both long (q).

Measurable disease. The use of an identified lesion that can be accurately measured in at least one dimension and be >10 mm when assessed by CT, MRI, or clinical examination; or >20 mm when measured by plain X-ray.

Metaplasia. The replacement of one differentiated cell type with another, often in response to persistent injury. It is reversible, such that removal of the stimulus can cause the cells to revert back to their original state.

Metastasis. The ability to proliferate in a distant part of the body after the cancer cells have migrated or been transported via the blood, lymphatics, or through body spaces.

Neoadjuvant chemotherapy. Chemotherapy administered first before a planned cytoreductive procedure. This can result in a reduced requirement for surgery, increase the likelihood of successful debulking, reduce the duration of hospitalisation and improve the fitness of the patient prior to interval debulking.

Neuropathic pain. Pain that arises from damage to nerves either peripherally or centrally, due to compression, ischaemia, haemorrhage, chemicals, or transection. Neuropathic pain is described as burning, shooting, stabbing, or 'pins and needles'.

Non-measurable disease. Includes aspects of the patient that are more subjective in their assessment and based on factors such as tumour marker levels, presence of ascites, or effusions.

Optimal dose distribution. A medical physicist or dosimetrist uses data from the radiotherapy simulation to determine the optimal dose distribution across the volume of the target tumour, while minimising the dose delivered to surrounding normal tissues. A complete collection of machine data, including depth dose and beam profile information, is calculated and this assists the radiation oncologist to decide the number of beams (usually two to four) and angles of entry. The goal is to maximise the dose to the tumour while minimising the dose to surrounding normal structures. Several treatment plans are often generated and the optimal dose distribution is selected by the radiation oncologist. The dose of radiation absorbed directly correlates with the energy of the radiation beam. An accurate measurement of the absorbed dose is therefore crucial in delivering radiotherapy treatments.

Overall survival rate. The percentage of patients in a study or treatment group who are alive for a certain period of time after the diagnosis of cancer, usually stated as a 5-year survival rate.

Palliative chemotherapy. Treatment primarily used to treat patients with metastasis. The goal is an improvement in symptoms with a focus on improving quality of life, and survival increments are secondary.

Parkinsonism. An adverse effect of metoclopramide, occurring days to weeks after starting the drug, producing rigidity and depression.

Partial remission. A state where some but not all of the signs and symptoms of cancer have disappeared.

Percentage depth dose. The dose of delivered radiation absorbed by target tissues can be measured and calculated to form a percentage depth dose curve. As the energy increases, the penetrative ability of the beam increases and the skin dose decreases.

Pleurectomy. A procedure that involves removal of some of the pleura. This results in obliteration of the pleural space and adhesion of the underlying tissues.

Pleurodesis. A procedure in which the pleural space is obliterated, usually by the instillation of an irritant substance that causes adhesion of the two layers of the pleura.

Pleuroperitoneal shunt. A tube structure that is surgically inserted between the pleural space and the peritoneal cavity. This facilitates drainage of pleural fluid into the abdomen to alleviate the symptoms of a pleural effusion.

Polyploidy. A cell with more than one complete chromosome set with multiples of the basic number of chromosomes characteristic of the species. In humans this would be 69, 92, etc.

Port films. For quality assurance of radiotherapy treatment, weekly images are generated by the linear accelerator at energies of 6–20 MeV. These ensure that the beams and blocks are consistently and correctly placed for each treatment.

Radiotherapy. The use of ionising radiation for therapeutic benefit. Can be by the use of external beam X-rays or radioisotopes that emit gamma or beta waves.

Remission rate. The percentage of patients who achieve a state where the cancer is no longer detectable.

Residual disease. The detectable disease that is left at completion of planned treatment. If present it indicates resistance to the treatment and is therefore an adverse prognostic factor. In some circumstances it may be difficult to distinguish residual disease from normal tissue, particularly in patients with postoperative changes following abdominal or pelvic surgery.

Response. The objective assessment of effectiveness of a particular treatment, usually assessed in accordance with the RECIST 1.1 criteria with pre-treatment documentation of target and non-target lesions.

Somatic pain. Pain that is commonly described as crushing, tearing and throbbing, and is usually well localised. It is transmitted via the spinothalamic tract which decussates at the level of the spinal cord, transmitting to the cortex via the thalamus, giving intensity and topographical location of the stimuli.

Stage. The extent of a cancer, usually using a defined classification, such as the TNM system, that is dependent on the primary site.

Systemic chemotherapy. Drug therapy administered to a patient that enters the circulation having been administered intravenously or orally.

Tardive dyskinesia. Repetitive involuntary movements, particularly around the mouth and tongue, often irreversible.

Translocation. The result of the reciprocal exchange of terminal segments of non-homologous chromosomes.

Treatment plan (radiotherapy). The planning computer calculates the data required for treatment, such as beam-on time, beam angles, blocks and wedges, and this data collection forms the treatment plan for the patient which is exported to the treatment machine. The therapy radiographer who actually treats the patient will use this information to set up and treat the patient consistently and accurately each day.

Visceral pain. Produces discomfort that is diffuse, poorly localised and is stimulated by chemical insult, ischaemia, inflammation, or compression or distension of organs.

Index

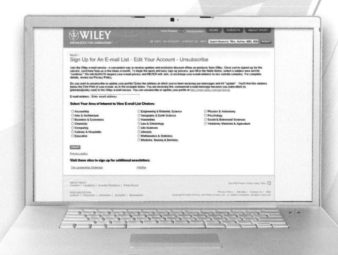
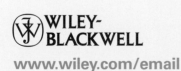

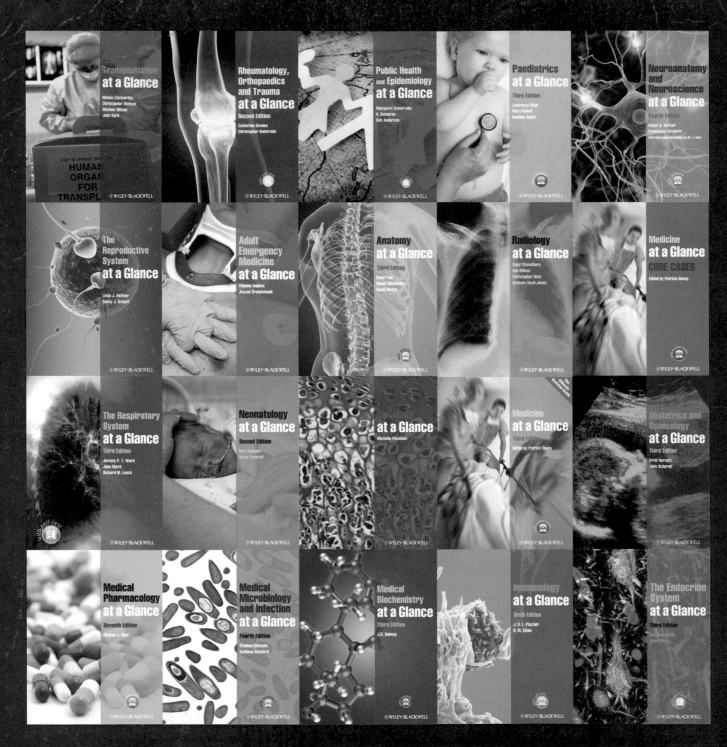

The at a Glance series

Popular double-page spread format • Coverage of core knowledge
Full-colour throughout • Self-assessment to test your knowledge • Expert authors

www.wileymedicaleducation.com

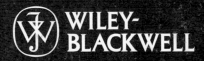

WILEY-BLACKWELL